CLINICAL GASTROENTEROLOGY

George Y. Wu, Series Editor

For other titles published in this series, go to
www.springer.com/series/7672

VIRAL HEPATITIS IN CHILDREN

UNIQUE FEATURES AND OPPORTUNITIES

Edited by

Maureen M. Jonas

Division of Gastroenterology, Children's Hospital Boston, Boston, MA, USA

Humana Press

Editor
Maureen M. Jonas
Division of Gastroenterology
Children's Hospital Boston
Harvard Medical School
Boston, MA, USA
maureen.jonas@childrens.harvard.edu

ISBN 978-1-60761-372-5 e-ISBN 978-1-60761-373-2
DOI 10.1007/978-1-60761-373-2
Springer New York Dordrecht Heidelberg London

Library of Congress Control Number: 2010934591

Printed on acid-free paper

Humana Press is part of Springer Science+Business Media (www.springer.com)

Preface

Acute and chronic viral hepatitis infections are serious public health threats around the world. The different infections have different epidemiology and natural histories, and children play important roles in each of these. For example, children are important reservoirs for acute hepatitis A, childhood infections are responsible for most of the global morbidity associated with chronic hepatitis B, and perinatal transmission of hepatitis C continues to occur, even as the overall incidence of new infections wanes. Some non-A through E viral hepatitis infections are seen predominantly in infants and young children, while others have specific implications for this population. Therapeutic options for children with chronic viral hepatitis are limited when compared to those available for adults, especially for hepatitis B, and considerations given to long-term therapy have dramatic implications when dealing with the long life expectancy of these young patients.

With these issues in mind, this unique volume has been created to address the special considerations regarding viral hepatitis in children. It includes the latest information and recommendations specifically directed at the pediatric population, and highlights the knowledge gaps which will need to be filled to improve our understanding of these infections and treatment of this special group. Experienced practitioners from around the world have contributed these reviews, incorporating the latest studies, the current recommendations, and the distinctive pediatric issues that shape clinical care, and will determine the research agenda for this field going forward. There is a chapter dedicated only to immunoprophylaxis, emphasizing the critical nature of this aspect of care in the important goals of control and eventual eradication of some of these infections. Another chapter is aimed specifically at the primary care issues that arise during evaluation and management of infants and children who are at risk for or affected by viral hepatitis. It is hoped that this work will be a valuable resource for pediatricians, pediatric gastroenterologists, and hepatologists and infectious disease specialists who may care for children with viral hepatitis.

Boston, MA　　　　　　　　　　　　　　　　　　　　Maureen M. Jonas

Contents

Contributors

Annemarie Broderick, MB, MMedSc, DCH, MRCPI (Paeds)
Consultant Paediatric Gastroenterologist, Our Lady's Children's Hospital, Crumlin, Dublin12, Ireland & UCD Senior Clinical Lecturer, School of Medicine and Medical Science, University College Dublin, Dublin 4, Ireland

Mei-Hwei Chang, MD
Department of Pediatrics, National Taiwan University Hospital, Taipei, Taiwan

Szu-Ta Chen, MD
Yun-Lin Branch, National Taiwan University Hospital, Taipei, Taiwan

Scott A. Elisofon, MD
Instructor in Pediatrics, Division of Gastroenterology and Nutrition, Children's Hospital Boston, Harvard Medical School, Boston MA, USA

Karan Emerick, MD
Division of Gastroenterology, Connecticut Children's Medical Center, Hartford CT, USA

Jessi Erlichman, MPH
Division of Gastroenterology, Hepatology, and Nutrition, The Children's Hospital of Philadelphia, Philadelphia PA, USA

Rima Fawaz, MD
Instructor in Pediatrics, Children's Hospital Boston, Boston MA, USA

Barbara A. Haber, MD
Associate Professor of Pediatrics, Division of Gastroenterology, Hepatology, and Nutrition, The Children's Hospital of Philadelphia, School of Medicine, University of Pennsylvania, Philadelphia PA, USA

Nanda Kerkar, MD
Associate Professor of Pediatrics and Surgery, Medical Director,
Pediatric Liver and Liver Transplant Program, Mount Sinai School of Medicine,
New York NY, USA

Will Mellman, MSW
Division of Gastroenterology, Hepatology, and Nutrition,
The Children's Hospital of Philadelphia, Philadelphia PA, USA

Karen F. Murray, MD
Director, Hepatobiliary Program Division of Gastroenterology and Hepatology,
Seattle Children's Hospital, Seattle WA, USA

Michelle Rook, MD
Fellow, Pediatric Gastroenterology, Hepatology and Nutrition,
Department of Pediatrics, University of California, San Francisco CA, USA

Philip Rosenthal, MD
Professor of Pediatrics and Surgery, Medical Director, Pediatric Liver
Transplantation Center, Director, Pediatric Hepatology,
University of California, San Francisco CA, USA

Hepatitis A in Children

Michelle Rook and Philip Rosenthal

Key Concepts

- Hepatitis A virus is the most common viral hepatitis globally.
- Hepatitis A virus is a serious public health concern, and causes significant morbidity and mortality.
- The changing epidemiological features of hepatitis A are associated with the inception of vaccine programs.
- Hepatitis A infection has numerous clinical presentations.

Keywords Hepatitis A • Epidemiology • Clinical manifestations • Prevention • Public health

Introduction

Hepatitis A virus (HAV), a non-enveloped ribonucleic acid (RNA) virus of the Picornaviridae family, was first detected by immune electron microscopy by Purcell in 1973. Globally, it is the most common form of viral hepatitis. It is transmitted via the fecal–oral route, spreading primarily through close individual contact, and has been the most common cause of acute hepatitis in the United States, and throughout the world. Due to advances in detection, prevention, and prophylaxis, infection with HAV has been on the decline. The development of accurate serologic tests has allowed for investigations into the epidemiology, clinical features, natural history, and rapid diagnosis of this disease.

M. Rook (✉)
Department of Pediatrics, University of California San Francisco, 500 Parnassus Avenue MU4E, San Francisco, CA 94108, USA
e-mail: rookm@peds.ucsf.edu

M.M. Jonas (ed.), *Viral Hepatitis in Children: Unique Features and Opportunities*, Clinical Gastroenterology, DOI 10.1007/978-1-60761-373-2_1,

Epidemiology

United States

Hepatitis A has been one of the most frequently reported infectious diseases, with an average of 28,000 cases per year reported between 1987 and 1997 [1]. The incidence of HAV in the United States reported by the CDC has declined 92% from 12 cases per 100,000 population in 1995 to 1.0 case per 100,000 in 2007, with the decline being the greatest in children [1]. There has been a drastic decrease in the reported cases of HAV (Table 1). The most recent data from 2007 suggest that acute symptomatic disease occurred in 2,979 individuals, with an estimation of 25,000 cases of asymptomatic disease and/or underreporting compared with 22,000–36,000 HAV cases reported annually from 1980 to 1995 [1, 2]. The lower incidence of HAV infections in the United States can most likely be attributed to the introduction of the hepatitis A vaccine in 1995 [1, 2].

Incidence of HAV infections in the United States varies based on geographic location, age, sex, race, and ethnicity [1]. The highest rates of HAV in the United States prior to 2002 were observed in western regions [1]. Prior to vaccination programs, the highest incidence of HAV occurred in children and young adults, and the lowest incidence in adults older than 40 years of age [1–3]. Current data demonstrate the reversal of these trends. During 2001–2007, the lowest incidence was found in children <5 years of age, and the highest incidence, 1.3 cases per 100,000 population, in adults 25–39 years of age [1]. Children <4 years of age typically are asymptomatic; therefore, there may be an underestimation of HAV in this specific population. Hepatitis A rates differed by race and ethnicity prior to 2007 [1, 4]. Highest rates were seen amongst American Indian, Alaskan natives, and Hispanics, with the lowest rates among Asian, Pacific Islanders and non-Hispanics [1]. Recently, there has been a uniform decline in the incidence of HAV amongst all ethnicities and races in the United States [1, 3, 4].

Table 1 Reported cases of HAV in the United States

Year	Number	Rate[a]
1970	56,797	27.9
1975	35,855	16.8
1980	29,087	12.8
1985	23,257	10
1990	31,441	12.6
1995	31,582	12
2000	13,582	4.8
2005	4,488	1.5
2007	2,979	1

[a]Rate per 100,000 population Adapted from Center for Disease Control [1]

Global

HAV has a global distribution, being the most common form of viral hepatitis worldwide. It is responsible for approximately 1.4 million new infections worldwide each year; however, the true incidence is often underestimated secondary to underreporting [5]. Endemic areas with the highest prevalence of seropositivity include Africa, Asia, South America, and the Middle East [5]. Japan, Australia, New Zealand, Canada, and the United States have the lowest seroprevalence [5]. Higher incidence and asymptomatic childhood infection are commonly associated with lower socioeconomic factors, overcrowding, poor sanitation, and inadequate water treatment [5]. Worldwide, three patterns of endemicity, low, intermediate, and high, are seen. In areas of high endemicity, more than 30–40% of children acquire HAV before 5 years of age, and almost all have been infected by early adulthood [5]. The reported disease incidence rate may reach 150 per 100,000 per year [5]. Areas of intermediate endemicity exist in developing countries, where there are transitional economies, and variability among sanitary conditions [5]. Regions in Southern and Eastern Europe and some regions in the Middle East have been identified as such areas. In areas of low endemicity, very few children become infected with HAV, leading them to be susceptible later in life [5, 6]. In areas with low HAV rates, specific risk groups, such as travelers, have been identified, in whom infection is more likely to occur [6].

Changes in the epidemiology of HAV have been recently observed in some parts of the world. This shift has been related to better hygiene and sanitation practices, and has modified the age distribution of seropositivity, from being highest in children to currently being highest in the adult population [5, 6]. In India, an area with high endemicity, the overall seroprevalence has been observed to be 65.9% [7]. Seropositivity increases with age from 52.2% in children 1–5 years of age to 80.8% in those greater than 16 years of age [7]. Here, no significant difference was observed between socioeconomic classes, but the highest seropositivity was associated with municipal water supplies [7]. In Egypt, the seroprevalence of HAV antibodies increases with age and is inversely proportional to social class [8]. In children less than 6 years of age, 72.7% of high and 10% of low social class were seronegative [8]. In a recent study from the Ukraine, an area with moderate HAV endemicity of 31.9%, anti-HAV seropositivity increased with age from 9.2% among children 1–5 years of age to 81.7% among adults greater than 50 years of age. This is consistent with the recent trends seen worldwide [9].

Mathematical models have been developed to assess the impact of socioeconomic factors on the seroprevalence patterns of HAV worldwide. Time-dependent infection rates, regional differences, and socioeconomic development for various age groups around the world have been evaluated [10, 11]. In one study, average annual infection rates were the highest in Africa, followed by the Americas, Middle East, and Asia, with rates in Europe being the lowest of all regions [10, 11]. In these models, significant independent predictors of infection have been found to be water sources, a human development index based on life expectancy, education, standard of living, and gross domestic product [10, 11]. Results of these mathematical models parallel the global endemicity.

Risk Factors

Recognizable risk factors among reported cases include close contact with an individual with HAV, international travel, household or personal contact with a child in daycare, food borne outbreak, male homosexual activity, and the use of illicit drugs (Table 1) [1]. In children less than 15 years of age, the most frequently known reported causes of disease are international travel, household contact with an individual infected with HAV, and a child or employee in a daycare center [1]. Approximately 10% of cases in the United States occur in daycare centers where children are not toilet trained [2]. Children in day care with an individual with hepatitis A are recommended to refrain from attending for approximately 1 week [3]. In the age group between 15 and 39 years of age, the most frequently known reported causes of HAV are international travel, contact with a hepatitis A patient, or suspected food or water borne outbreak [1]. Most cases in both age groups have no identifiable risk factors. HAV is transmitted via the fecal–oral route, often from asymptomatic children.

The Virus

HAV is a single-stranded RNA virus. Infectivity occurs primarily through fecal-oral transmission and, after ingestion and absorption, the virus replicates in the liver and is excreted in bile. HAV enters into the hepatocyte by specific receptors located on the plasma membrane. Viral RNA is encoated after uptake and binds to ribosomes, stimulating the synthesis of viral proteins, and replication of the viral genome occurs by RNA polymerase. The virus is then secreted into the biliary tree and excreted in feces, where high concentrations of HAV are detected [12, 13]. An immunologic response occurs within the liver, leading to portal and periportal lymphocytic infiltration, and potentiates liver damage. A limited number of cases have been reported from blood transfusions, and vertical transmission from mother to fetus.

Transmission of HAV is the highest during the anicteric prodrome of 14–21 days, when fecal and serum virus concentrations are high [2, 12, 13]. The incubation period is typically 2–6 weeks, with an average of 28 days. Fecal viral excretion may persist for up to 3 weeks. Immunoglobulins to HAV (IgM anti-HAV antibodies) can first be detected in serum 5–10 days after exposure, and are diagnostic of acute infection when detected (Table 2). Commercially available assays

Table 2 Clinical features of HAV infection

Week	Symptoms	Laboratory features
0–3	Flu-like illness	Fecal HAV
		IgM anti-HAV
2–12	Flu-like illness	IgM anti-HAV
	Jaundice	Elevated aminotransferases
	Dark urine	Hyperbilirubinemia
		+/– IgG anti-HAV
>12	Cholestatic	IgM anti-HAV
		Elevated aminotransferases
		Hyperbilirubinemia
		+/– IgG anti-HAV

for anti-HAV IgM are extremely accurate, with a positive predictive value of 88% within the first 2 weeks of infection [2]. IgM anti-HAV antibodies will peak by 10 weeks after exposure, when clinical symptoms appear, and become undetectable less than 6 months after infection [2, 12, 13]. Thus, the presence of IgM anti-HAV antibodies indicates recent or current infection. IgG anti-HAV antibodies become detectable in serum shortly after the appearance of IgM anti-HAV antibodies, and represent past infection and immunity.

HAV is resistant to denaturation by acid substances with a pH of greater than 3.0, ether, drying, and can sustain temperatures between –20°C and 56°C. Inactivation of HAV occurs by treatment at temperatures greater than 185°F, or with formalin or chlorine.

Clinical Features

Acute hepatitis A is an acute illness with virus-like symptoms and jaundice and/or elevated serum aminotransferases. Initial clinical manifestations may be those of a viral prodrome, with nonspecific symptoms such as nausea, vomiting, anorexia, fatigue, weight loss, low grade fevers, myalgia, arthralgia, and headaches. Individuals remain in this anicteric phase for an average of 7 days [2, 12, 13]. Progression to the icteric phase commences with dark urine secondary to excretion of bilirubin, and may be followed by pale stools. Jaundice is present in only 10% of children less than 6 years of age, 40% of children between 6 and 14 years of age, and 70% of children greater than 14 years of age, compared to 70–85% of adults [1, 2, 12, 13]. Risk of transmission decreases 1 week after the onset of jaundice. Additional symptoms may include abdominal pain, pruritis, arthralgias, rash, fever, and hepatomegaly. The duration of symptoms is several weeks in typical disease, with a mean of 4 weeks, and may be directly correlated to the viral load of HAV. Resolution is spontaneous, with typically minimal sequelae.

Diagnosis

Diagnosis of acute HAV is confirmed by the detection of IgM anti-HAV antibodies. Appropriate additional evaluation includes evaluation of serum IgG anti-HAV antibodies, alanine aminotransferase (ALT), aspartate aminotransferase (AST), alkaline phosphatase, total bilirubin (TB), direct bilirubin (DB), albumin, total protein, coagulation profiles, and complete blood count (CBC). Elevated serum ALT is correlated with the inception of HAV, and is present when individuals are symptomatic. ALT is often greater than AST, with levels 20–100 times the upper limit of normal [2]. Asymptomatic children with elevations in ALT and in contact with an index case should be tested for HAV. Variability exists, as serum transaminases may normalize within approximately 3 weeks or remain elevated for several months. Serum bilirubin levels rise with the onset of jaundice, peak at approximately 10 mg/dL, and usually normalize within 4 weeks [2, 12, 13]. Persistent elevation in serum bilirubin is suspicious for cholestatic hepatitis. Serum lipid profiles, including triglyceride, cholesterol, low-density lipoprotein (LDL), and high-density lipoprotein (HDL) may have important implications [14]. There are limited data in children showing elevated serum triglycerides at the onset of acute HAV. After recovery, serum triglycerides, cholesterol, and LDL decreased, while HDL increased in the same population [14].

More data on the clinical significance of lipid profiles are necessary prior to their use as routine testing. Additional laboratory evaluation may be useful in determining synthetic hepatic function and evaluating alternative etiologies of liver disease if suspicious.

Children may serve as a reservoir for transmission of HAV. They are often undiagnosed because of a lack of jaundice, and their symptoms mimic typical viral illness such as gastroenteritis. In one study, 57% of adults without a known source of infection had a child less than 6 years of age in the household [6].

Atypical HAV

Atypical manifestations of HAV have been recognized, and are associated with persistence of IgM anti-HAV antibodies for as long as 6–12 months [2]. Cholestatic hepatitis, relapsing hepatitis, immune complex disorders, autoimmune hepatitis, and other rare disease processes have been associated with HAV (Table 3). Prolonged jaundice greater than 12 weeks associated with pruritis, fever, diarrhea, and weight loss with serum bilirubin levels greater than 10 mg/dL is a feature of cholestatic hepatitis [2]. Cholestatic hepatitis may persist for several months prior to spontaneous resolution. Treatment with ursodeoxycholic acid may be helpful for symptomatic relief of pruritis, and may aid in improving cholestasis. The frequency of this form of HAV infection increases with age. Treatment with corticosteroids may be effective in reducing the duration of cholestatic hepatitis; however, there is

Table 3 Atypical presentations of HAV infection

Cholestatic hepatitis
Relapsing hepatitis
Immune complex disorders
Autoimmune disease
Wilson disease
Aplastic Anemia
Hemophagocytic syndrome
Thrombocytopenic purpura
Acute renal failure
Pancreatitis
Guillan–Barré syndrome
Transient heart block
Autoimmune hepatitis
Acute liver failure

minimal literature documenting full resolution, and immunosuppression with steroids may lead to reactivation of HAV.

Relapsing HAV occurs in 3–20% of infected individuals and each relapse resembles the initial presentation [2, 15]. It is characterized by an initial episode of acute hepatitis with remission lasting 4–15 weeks, and may become a cyclic process over 3–9 months with episodes of remission in between relapsing periods [2, 15]. Symptoms are typically mild, but worse with more severe cholestasis. Viral shedding persists. A high fecal HAV viral load and IgM anti-HAV antibodies are present [16].

HAV has been associated with immune complex disorders, including cutaneous vasculitis, arthritis, cryoglobulinemia, lupus-like syndromes, and Sjögren syndrome [2]. Other rare complications include acute renal failure, interstitial nephritis, pancreatitis, anemia, bone marrow suppression, transient heart block, and Guillain–Barré syndrome [2, 17]. Acute HAV has been reported as a trigger in the presentation of autoimmune hepatitis and Wilson disease [2, 18]. Chronic infection is not seen with HAV. Protective antibodies which confer lifelong immunity develop in response to acute HAV. Fulminant hepatitis is rare in the US, but may be seen in those with underlying liver disease.

Although uncommon in the US, HAV has been determined to be a major cause of acute liver failure (ALF) in children and adolescents in Latin America, Asia, and Europe [19, 20]. Every child presenting in ALF should have serological testing. In a recent prospective, multicenter study in Latin American children and adolescents, 43% of those with ALF were positive for IgM anti-HAV immunoglobulin, indicating that HAV was the primary etiologic agent, and 73% of those were children 3–5 years of age [19]. In prior studies, HAV-associated ALF was found to account for 64% of cases in Argentina, 71% in Chile, and 82% in Brazil [19]. HAV was found to be the etiology of pediatric ALF in 38–50% of cases in South Africa, India, Pakistan, and Argentina [19]. HAV-associated ALF is not benign, and up to 45% of patients will require transplantation [19, 20].

Treatment

HAV is a self-limited disease, and treatment includes only supportive measures in uncomplicated cases. Treatment is targeted at specific symptoms; bed rest is recommended, and increased fluid intake is necessary to prevent dehydration in the case of emesis and diarrhea [2, 3]. Intravenous fluids may be necessary depending on the severity of illness. Children with HAV infection usually have milder symptoms than adults. Identifying the index case is warranted to prevent spread of disease. Individuals should be advised to refrain from returning to work for approximately 10 days, and children with HAV or in contact with an index case should be out of day care or school for a minimum of 1 week [2, 3]. In practice, it may be prudent to limit medications that are hepatotoxic, and acetaminophen use should be cautiously monitored in children with acute hepatitis due to HAV to limit potential complications; however, there are no official guidelines present at this time.

In cases in which HAV acts as a trigger for secondary disorders, including autoimmune hepatitis and Wilson disease, treatment should target the specific disease process in a timely fashion. HAV results in 3–8% of fulminant hepatic failure [19]. Children with this complication should be monitored for encephalopathy, hypoglycemia, coagulopathy, renal failure, and cerebral edema. Early referral to a transplant center may be necessary.

Prevention

Prevention measures are recommended in communities and hospital settings. Improvements in sanitation, water sources, and food preparation have decreased the spread of HAV. Personal hygiene, hand washing, and proper disposal of diapers in child-care settings can reduce transmission. The primary goal is prevention of the spread of HAV by basic measures. Secondary goals include immunoprophylaxis and immunization to decrease the incidence and shorten the outbreaks of HAV, and to induce development of herd immunity in populations.

Travelers to endemic areas should avoid possible contaminated water sources, raw shellfish, and uncooked foods. HAV is inactivated by boiling water or by adding iodine.

Immunoprophylaxis

Immunoprophylaxis of HAV infection is discussed in detail in Chap. 8. Post-exposure prophylaxis is recommended for children greater than 12 months of age. HAV vaccine is recommended as soon as possible after exposure for those between 12 months and 40 years of age. Immune globulin is preferred for adults greater than

40 years of age. Immunoprophylaxis with intramuscular immune globulin is 85% effective when given within 2 weeks after HAV exposure. If immune globulin cannot be obtained, HAV vaccine should be given.

Travelers to areas with endemic HAV should receive pre-exposure prophylaxis. Children less than 12 months of age should receive immune globulin 0.02 mL/kg. For travel greater than 3 months, 0.06 mL/kg is recommended, and then repeated every 5 months if there is exposure to HAV. Travelers aged 12 months to 40 years should receive the hepatitis A vaccine.

Vaccination Implications

The incidence of HAV in the US has declined drastically with the introduction of the HAV vaccine in 1995. Prior to 1995, cyclic patterns of HAV included increased rates every 10–15 years. In 1999 the Advisory Committee on Immunization Practices (ACIP) of the American Academy of Pediatrics recommended routine vaccination for children in 11 states with HAV rates of 20 cases per 100,000 population, twice the national average, between 1987 and 1997. Implementation of this recommendation resulted in a greater decline in HAV rates in states participating in such vaccination programs than that in states not participating. Routine vaccination was also implemented at that time in six states where the annual rates were between 10 and 20 cases per 100,000 population. In 2006, universal HAV vaccine recommendations were made to include all children aged 12–23 months in all 50 states. HAV infection rates in all regions of the US have declined significantly due to the implementation of these recommendations.

The age distribution of persons with HAV has changed with the implementation of universal vaccine programs. Children aged 5–14 years had the highest incidence of HAV in the pre-vaccine era, but males aged 20–39 years were the highest incidence group in 2007. Approximately 30% of the US population had evidence of immunity to HAV as evidenced by data from the Third National Health and Nutrition Examination Survey (NHANES III) during 1988–1994.

Racial and ethnic differences no longer exist in the post-vaccine era. Use of the HAV vaccine began in 1996 in Native American communities, and their rates now equal those of other races/ethnicities. Rates for Hispanics are currently similar to those for non-Hispanics, and declined drastically from 1997 to 2007 from 24.1 cases per 100,000 population to 1.4 cases per 100,000 population.

Public Health Implications

HAV infection imposes a considerable economic burden throughout the world, and causes significant morbidity and mortality. HAV-related costs in the United States were recently estimated to be between one and three million dollars annually.

Costs include outpatient care, inpatient care, fulminant liver failure, and liver transplants due to this disease. On average, infected adults miss approximately 30 days of work. In the US, HAV is a reportable infectious disease, increasing the public health costs. Case reporting of HAV increases public health surveillance, contact tracing, and outbreak response, including prophylaxis and prevention measures to be taken once a case of HAV is identified. Routine childhood vaccine programs can drastically decrease the public health costs in the United States and globally by decreasing the worldwide incidence of HAV infection. Cost-effective analyses have clearly demonstrated the benefit of vaccination programs. One model has estimated the total economic costs associated with HAV to be 133.5 million dollars based on a 2005 birth cohort, including 86.8 million dollars in health care and adult vaccination costs, 31.6 million dollars in work-related losses to parents of infected children, and 15.3 million dollars in work-related losses to infected adults. Models have been adapted to examine the effects of implementing the HAV vaccine-related cost effectiveness, and have demonstrated that there is reduction in disease events, medical services, total healthcare costs, and work-related losses.

Current Trends

HAV infection continues to be one of the most frequently reported vaccine-preventable diseases, even with the most recent CDC and ACIP recommendations [4]. Community wide outbreaks still occur throughout the United States, indicating that HAV remains a public health threat [6]. The decline in the incidence of HAV is most attributable to improved hygiene and sanitation; however, it does remain underreported as most children are asymptomatic. Despite the reversed epidemiological trends in reporting HAV, the importance of universal routine childhood vaccination programs on a global level should be stressed. The availability of a safe and effective HAV vaccine provides the opportunity to substantially lower the incidence of disease; potentially eradicate infection; and offset the morbidity, mortality and healthcare costs associated with this vaccine preventable disease [6].

References

1. CDC. Surveillance for acute viral hepatitis – United States 2007. MMWR. 2009;58:1–32. http://cdc.gov/mmwr
2. Denson LA. Postnatal Infections, Part 1C: Other Viral Infections. In: Walker WA. Pediatric Gastroenterology Disease: Pathophysiology, Diagnosis, Management. 4th Ed. Hamilton, ON:BC Decker; 2004:1170–1178
3. Koslap-Petraco MB, Shub M, Judelsohn R; Hepatitis A: Disease burden and current childhood vaccination strategies in the United States. J Pediatr Health Care. 2008;22:3–11
4. CDC. Prevention of hepatitis A through active or passive immunization: Recommendations of the Advisory Committee on Immunization Practices (ACIP). MMWR Recomm Rep. 2006;55:1–23

5. World Health Organization. Hepatitis A Surveillance and Control. http://www.who.int/csr/disease/hepatitis/whocdscsredc2007/en/index4.html. Accessed Dec 16 2009.
6. Rosenthal P; Hepatitis A: A preventable threat. J Pediatr Gastroenterol Nutr. 2002;35:595–596
7. Mall ML, Rai RR, Philip M, et al; Seroprevalence of hepatitis A infection in India: Changing pattern. Indian J Gastroenterol. 2001;20:132–135
8. Al-Aziz AM, Award MA; Seroprevalence of hepatitis A virus antibodies among a sample of Egyptian children. East Mediterr Health J. 2008;14(5):1028–1035
9. Moisseeva AV, Marichev IL, Biloschitchkay NA, et al; Hepatitis A seroprevalence in children and adults in Kiev City, Ukraine. J Viral Hepat. 2008;15:43–46
10. Jacobsen KH, Koopman JS; The effects of socioeconomic development on worldwide hepatitis A virus seroprevalence patterns. Int J Epidemiol. 2005;34:600–609
11. Jacobsen KH, Koopman JS; Declining hepatitis A seroprevalence: A global review and analysis. Epidemiol Infect. 2004;132:1005–1022
12. Leach C; Hepatitis A in the United States. Pediatr Infect Dis J. 2004;23:551–552
13. Dentinger C; Emerging Infections: Hepatitis A. Am J Nurs. 2009;109:29–33
14. Selimoglu MA, Caner I, Yildiz L; Lipid Profile in children with acute viral hepatitis A. Pediatr Int. 2007;49:215–219
15. Rachima CM, Cohen E, Garty M; Acute Hepatitis A: combination of relapsing and the cholestatic forms, two rare variants. Am J Med Sci. 2000;319:417–419
16. Sjogren MH, Tanno H, Sileoni S, et al; Hepatitis A virus in stool during clinical relapse. Ann Intern Med. 1997;106(2):221–226
17. Chatzmichael A, Schoina M, Arvanitidou V, et al; Hematologic complications of Hepatitis A: Another reason for implemenatation of anti-HAV vaccination. J Pediatr Hematol Oncol. 2008;30:562
18. Ozcay F, Canan O, Akcan B, et al; Hepatitis A super infection as a cause of liver failure in a child with Wilson's disease. Turk J Pediatr. 2007;49:199–202
19. Ciocca M, Moreira-Silva SF, Alegria S, et al; Hepatitis A as an etiologic agent of acute liver failure in Latin America. Pediatr Infect Dis J. 2007;26:711–715
20. Yeung L, Roberts EA; Current issues in the management of paediatric viral hepatitis. Liver Int. 2009;30(1):5–18

Epidemiology and Natural History of Hepatitis B in Children

Szu-Ta Chen and Mei-Hwei Chang

Key Concepts

- Patients in countries with high HBV endemicity tend to have perinatal transmission of hepatitis B, whereas those in countries with low endemicity have horizontal infection in adolescence or early adulthood.
- Universal infant immunization could effectively reduce the prevalence of HBV infection to approximately 10% of the prevalence before the vaccination program.
- Important factors affecting HBsAg seroconversion included maternal HBeAg status, virus genotypes, and host effects.

Keywords Epidemiology • Acute hepatitis B • Chronic hepatitis B • Fulminant hepatitis B • Hepatocellular carcinoma • Hepatitis B e seroconversion

Introduction

Hepatitis B virus (HBV) infection is a worldwide health problem and may lead to acute, fulminant, or chronic hepatitis; liver cirrhosis; and hepatocellular carcinoma (HCC) [1]. Approximately two billion people in the world have been infected by HBV, and 350 million of them are chronically infected, with a 25% of mortality risk related to the sequelae of hepatitis B. Roughly, an estimated one million deaths annually are attributed to HBV infection [2, 3]. Therefore, the burden of HBV infection is huge, and understandings of the natural history of HBV infection are extremely important to design preventive and therapeutic strategies.

M.-H. Chang (✉)
Department of Pediatrics, National Taiwan University Hospital,
No. 7, Chung-Shan S. Road, Taipei, Taiwan
e-mail: changmh@ntu.edu.tw

M.M. Jonas (ed.), *Viral Hepatitis in Children: Unique Features and Opportunities*,
Clinical Gastroenterology, DOI 10.1007/978-1-60761-373-2_2,

Epidemiology of Hepatitis B Virus Infection in Children Before the Era of Immunization Programs

Global

The prevalence of HBV infection varies in different countries or regions in the world (Fig. 1) as well as in different ethnic groups. HBV endemicity has been classified into three categories, high (>8%), intermediate (2–8%), and low (<2%), depending on the prevalence of hepatitis B surface antigen (HBsAg) seropositivity. The highly endemic areas in the world include East and Southeast Asia, the Pacific, sub-Saharan Africa, and parts of southern Europe. In North America, and western and northern Europe, HBV infection is relatively rare, with a prevalence rate of around 0.1%.

North America

Overall, the prevalence of HBV infection in this region is low. In the United States, the Third National Health and Nutrition Examination Survey (NHANES III), conducted from 1988 to 1994, revealed that the HBsAg seropositive rate was 0.41%, and the prevalence of previous or current HBV infection, i.e., seropositive antibodies against hepatitis B core antigen (anti-HBc), declined from 5.5 to 4.9%,

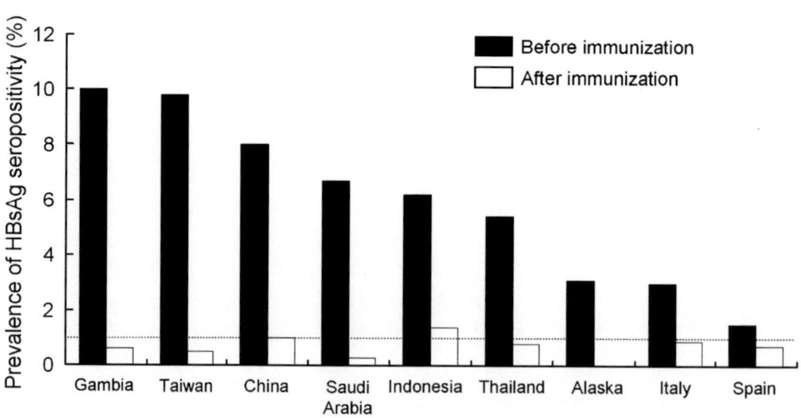

Fig. 1 Epidemiology of chronic hepatitis B in children before and after universal infant immunization programs [4–14]. All infants received three or four doses of HBV vaccine. Besides, hepatitis B immunoglobulin (HBIG) is given to infants of positive maternal HBsAg and HBeAg status (Taiwan [5] and China [10, 11]); or to infants of positive maternal HBsAg status (the United States [4], Italy [8], Spain [9], etc.) within 24 h after birth. The HBsAg seropositive rates declined to below 1% (*dotted line*) in most countries after hepatitis B immunization, regardless of the endemicity before vaccination. (*HBsAg* hepatitis B surface antigen; *HBeAg* hepatitis B e antigen)

compared to the results from NHANES II in 1976–1980 [15]. The prevalence of HBV infection in both NHANES studies was low in children upto 12 years of age and increased thereafter in all ethnic groups. After the 1991 recommendation for universal hepatitis B vaccination in the United States, the incidence of acute hepatitis B among children has declined in all ethnic groups to 0.3 cases per 100,000 in 2002 [16]. In Alaska, 10 years after institution of the routine immunization program, the prevalence of resolved HBV infection by 9 years of age declined from 7.6 to 1.5%; the HBsAg-seropositive prevalence also declined from 3.1 to 0% [4].

In Canada, the prevalence of HBsAg seropositivity through the National Notifiable Disease Reporting (NNDR) system is estimated to be 0.5–1.0% of the population [17]. Most acute HBV infections are associated with injection drug use and heterosexual activities. Mother-to-infant transmission is not a major route of HBV acquisition in Canada. Nevertheless, infant routine vaccination strategies have successfully decreased hepatitis B carriage in North America [18].

Europe

The HBsAg seroprevalence in this region varies widely, ranging from 0.3 to 12%, even within a single country [19]. The most frequently reported risk factors for hepatitis B in Europe include heterosexual activity, injection drug use, male homosexual activity, perinatal exposure, and household contact with infected individuals [20]. By the end of 2002, 41 of the 51 countries of the World Health Organization European Region had implemented universal hepatitis B vaccination programs for infants or adolescents [21]. The universal vaccination program was introduced in Italy in 1991; population surveys in 1994–1995 showed a significant decline in hepatitis B prevalence and a 50% reduction in acute hepatitis B incidence [22]. Some very low prevalence countries, such as Denmark, Finland, Iceland, Ireland, Federal republic of Yugoslavia, Netherland, Norway, Sweden, and United Kingdom, do not yet incorporate universal HBV vaccination for economic reasons.

Asia-Pacific Region

This area has countries with the highest prevalence level of endemic HBV infection (>8% HBsAg positivity) in the world, such as China, South Korea, Taiwan, Thailand and Vietnam [23]. Some countries in this area, such as Japan, Australia, and New Zealand, have low HBsAg prevalence rates. In the high endemic areas, perinatal infection and household contact with chronically infected patients during early childhood are the predominant modes of transmission [23]. For example, in Taiwan, before the implementation of a universal HBV immunization program, the HBsAg seropositivity rate of children in highly endemic areas was 5% in infants and increased to 10% at 2 years of age, remaining at the same rate thereafter. However, the anti-HBc antibody seropositivity rate reached 50% by the age of 15 years. This suggests that most HBsAg carriers in this population were infected before 2 years of age due to perinatal or early childhood transmission [5, 24]. In low prevalence areas, HBV infection is acquired mainly in adolescents and adults. Childhood HBV infection in this population is concentrated in immigrants from hyperendemic areas and in high-risk groups, such as children of intravenous drug users.

Africa

After Asia, Africa has the second largest number of individuals with chronic HBV infection, approaching 58 million [25]. Although overall Africa is considered a high endemic area with 7–26% prevalence of HBsAg, Tunisia, Morocco, and Zambia have intermediate endemicity [26]. In some countries in western Africa, e.g., Senegal and Gambia, over 90% of the population are exposed to and become infected with HBV during their lives [27]. Because of high HBV endemicity, Gambia was the first country in Africa to implement a mass infant immunization program in 1990, and demonstrated a reduced HBV burden in children, with HBsAg prevalence decreasing from 10.0 to 0.6% [6, 7]. In contrast to Asia, where mother-to-infant transmission is an important route, horizontal transmission in early life is considered to be the predominant mode of transmission in most of sub-Saharan Africa [28]. In rural areas of west Africa, HBV infection rates increase rapidly from the age of 6 months, and by the age of 2 years, 40% of children are infected and 15% develop chronic infection. By the age of 10 years, 90% of children become infected and 20% are chronic carriers [29].

HBV Transmission in Children

Major routes of HBV transmission include perinatal infection, horizontal infection, sexual behaviors, and intravenous drugs use. The transmission patterns differ in countries according to HBV endemicity. In hyperendemic areas, perinatal and horizontal infections in childhood are responsible for most transmission of infection; in intermediate endemic areas, a mix of various routes of transmission are observed; and in low endemic countries, most new infections occur in young adults through sexual intercourse or injecting drugs. Perinatal transmission from HBsAg-positive mothers to their infants is an important route of transmission in children (Table 1), and accounts for 40–50% before and 90% after the HBV vaccination era of HBsAg carriers in endemic areas in Asia such as Taiwan [5]. The young age of HBV infection and maternal hepatitis B e antigen (HBeAg) seropositivity are important factors in determining chronicity in children [30–33]. Chronic HBV infection develops in 90% of infected neonates or infants but only in 1–5% of

Table 1 Outcome of HBV infection in infants with different immunoprophylaxis strategies and maternal HBeAg status

HBsAg (+) mother	Infant		
	No vaccination	Vaccination	HBIG + vaccination
HBeAg (+)	>90% chronic infection	20–25% chronic infection [30]	10–15% chronic infection
HBeAg (−)	<5% chronic infection	<1% chronic infection	<1% chronic infection [31]

HBeAg hepatitis B e antigen; *HBsAg* hepatitis B surface antigen; *HBIG* hepatitis B immunoglobulin

infected adults [34]. Approximately 90% of the infants of HBeAg-positive mothers become HBsAg carriers without HBV immunization, regardless of whether the HBsAg carrier rate in the population is high or low [35]. Although HBV is found in breast milk, breast feeding is permitted for the mother who is infected with hepatitis B, since this has not been implicated in transmission. It is widely accepted that most perinatal transmissions occur at or near the time of birth, since neonatal vaccination prevents newborn infection in about 80–95% of cases. Theoretical risks for HBV transmission at delivery include exposure to cervical secretions and maternal blood. Transplacental (intrauterine) transmission is presumed to cause the minority of infections not prevented by prompt immunization. An observational study from Taiwan described a lower (9.7%) transmission rate to infants of highly infectious mothers delivered after cesarean section in comparison to a higher (24.9%) rate of transmission after vaginal delivery [36]. Another study compared outcomes among three groups: 144 infants born by spontaneous vaginal delivery, 40 by forceps or vacuum extraction, and 117 by cesarean section [37]. All infants received HBIG and HBV vaccine at the recommended schedule. Chronic HBV infection was detected in the infants in 7.3, 7.7, and 6.8%, respectively, and response rates to immunization were similar in all groups. The authors concluded that mode of delivery does not influence the likelihood of HBV transmission. The effects of different modes of delivery have not been confirmed, and routine cesarean section is not recommended.

The Effect of HBV Immunization in Children and Adolescents

Universal hepatitis B vaccination programs in some hyperendemic countries have effectively reduced the prevalence rate and reduce the chronic HBV infection rate (Fig. 1). Countries or regions that were examples of early implementation of universal HBV immunization include Taiwan (1984), Hong Kong (1988), Israel (1989), Malaysia (1990), Gambia (1990), Italy (1991), Spain (1991), and the United States (1991).

Strategies of HBV immunization vary in different countries depending on the seroepidemiologic status and the resources of the countries (Table 2). All infants receive three or four doses of HBV vaccine in the universal HBV vaccination

Table 2 Examples of different strategies for universal hepatitis B immunization in infants [9]

		Infants		
Maternal screening	Maternal status	Vaccine	HBIG	Example
HBsAg and HBeAg	HBsAg+, HBeAg+	Yes	Yes	Taiwan
	HBsAg+, HBeAg−	Yes	No	
HBsAg	HBsAg+	Yes	Yes	United States
	HBsAg−	Yes	No	
No	Unknown	Yes	No	Thailand

HBIG hepatitis B immunoglobulin; *HBsAg* hepatitis B surface antigen; *HBeAg* hepatitis B e antigen

program. Besides, hepatitis B immunoglobulin (HBIG) is given within 24 h after birth to infants of HBsAg- and HBeAg-positive mothers in some countries such as Taiwan [5], or to infants of HBsAg-positive mothers in the United States [4], Italy [8], Spain [9], etc. In countries with limited resources, maternal screening is not performed and no HBIG is given [38].

Taiwan has the longest experience with HBV immunization in the world, and has been a good example of a highly endemic area with a striking reduction in the burden of hepatitis B infection resulting from universal infant vaccination. HBsAg seroprevalence among Taiwanese children declined from 9.8% in 1984 to 0.5% in 2004 [5]; this universal vaccination program is poised to change Taiwan from a hyperendemic country to a low endemic country in the coming years. The HBsAg seropositivity rates declined to below 1% in most countries worldwide after universal infant hepatitis B immunization, regardless of the endemicity before vaccination [4–14] (Fig. 1).

Moreover, universal infant HBV immunization may reduce the incidence of HCC in childhood and early adulthood. The average annual incidence of HCC in Taiwanese children aged 6–14 years decreased from 0.52 to 0.54 cases per 100,000 children of the birth cohort born before the HBV vaccination program, to 0.13–0.20 cases in those born after the HBV vaccination program ($P<0.01$) [39–41]. According to a 20-year follow-up study of national cancer surveillance in Taiwan, prevention of HCC by universal HBV vaccination was observed not only in children but also extended to adolescents, with an age- and sex-adjusted relative risk of 0.31 for persons vaccinated at birth [42]. HBV vaccine is the first human vaccine demonstrated to prevent the development of cancer. In addition to the beneficial effects on prevalence of HBV infection and incidence of HCC, after the universal vaccination program was instituted, the mortality rate of fulminant hepatitis among Taiwanese infants declined by 68% [43, 44].

Natural History of Hepatitis B Virus Infection in Children

Primary HBV infection can lead to acute hepatitis, fulminant hepatitis, or chronic infection under different conditions (Fig. 2). The interaction between virus and host determines the outcome of HBV infection.

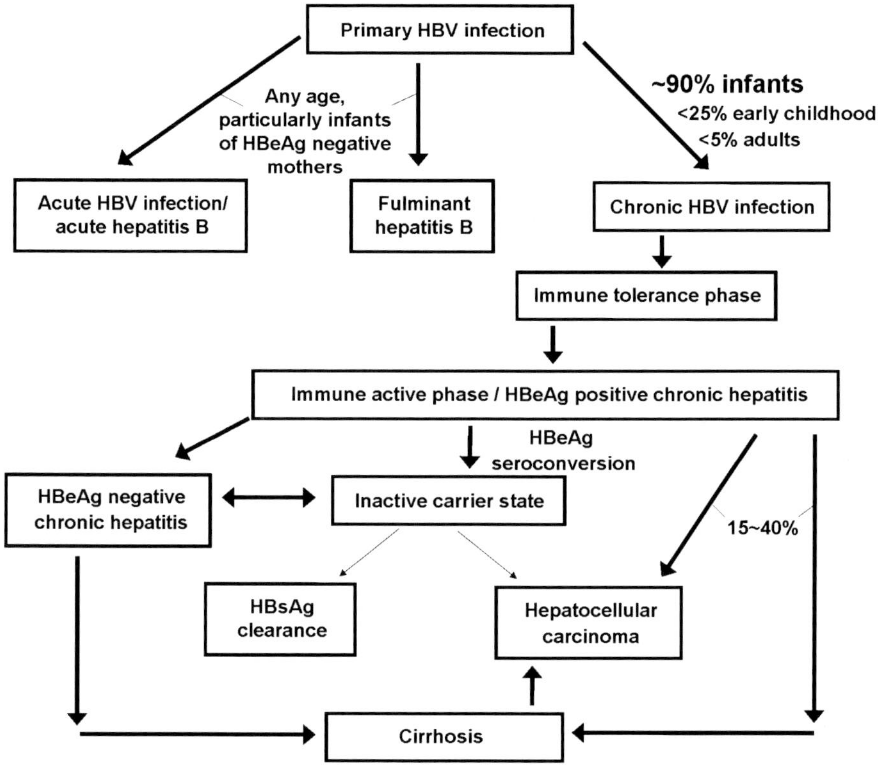

Fig. 2 Clinical courses of primary HBV infection. The rate of chronicity after primary HBV infection differs with the age of infection, implying a lower chronicity rate as the age of infection increases. (*HBV* hepatitis B virus; *HBeAg* hepatitis B e antigen)

Acute HBV Infection

Acute HBV infection in children can be either symptomatic or asymptomatic; the latter is more common, especially in infants and young children. Acute infection runs a self-limited course and recovery is marked by hepatitis B surface antibody (anti-HBs) seroconversion. In symptomatic patients, the prodromal symptoms, including general malaise, anorexia, nausea, vomiting, and fever, may persist for several days to weeks. Some cases may have jaundice with or without light yellow stool. Hepatomegaly with tenderness on right upper quadrant of abdomen is typical; however, splenomegaly is uncommon. Alanine aminotransferase (ALT) levels do not increase until after viral infection is well established because time is required for virus-specific cytotoxic T lymphocytes to develop against HBV-infected hepatocytes.

In acute hepatitis B, HBsAg is the first marker detectable in the blood after an incubation period of 4–10 weeks, followed shortly by anti-HBc antibodies, which are predominantly of the IgM type in the early phase. Viremia is established by the time HBsAg is detected, and the level of HBV DNA in acute infection is very high, frequently in the range of 10^9–10^{12} copies/mL (10^8–10^{11} IU/mL). Circulating HBeAg can be detected early but is cleared rapidly in patients with acute hepatitis B, and anti-HBs antibodies appear within 6 months of disease onset in most patients.

Patients with acute hepatitis B usually recover completely from the liver damage with the development of lasting immunity to reinfection. However, with the development of sensitive assays for HBV DNA, it has been determined that low levels of HBV DNA may persist in the blood for up to 10 years in some patients, despite the presence of anti-HBs and specific cytotoxic T lymphocytes [45]. These observations suggest that HBV may not be completely eradicated after recovery from acute hepatitis, which supports reports of reactivation of HBV replication in patients with anti-HBs who receive chemotherapy or immunosuppression after organ transplantation [46].

Fulminant Hepatitis B

Fulminant hepatitis B should be considered in children who develop signs of liver failure, including coagulopathy, increasing bilirubin levels with declining aminotransferase levels, and a decreasing liver size, with or without hepatic encephalopathy, within 8 weeks after the initial symptoms of HBV [47]. Bernuau and colleagues defined fulminant hepatitis as hepatic encephalopathy developing 2 weeks after the onset of jaundice and subfulminant hepatitis as hepatic encephalopathy developing between 2 and 12 weeks after the onset of jaundice [48]. The incidence of fulminant hepatitis B is higher in infancy than in other age periods [43]. As the diagnosis of hepatic encephalopathy is difficult to establish in infants aged less than 1 year, the presence of hepatic encephalopathy is not an absolute requisite for fulminant hepatic failure in this age group [47, 49]. Fulminant hepatitis B can occur as early as 2 months of age in infants of HBsAg-positive mothers [43]. Maternal transmission is the most important route in infants with fulminant hepatitis B, especially in those of HBeAg seronegative mothers [50]. The mortality rate for infants with fulminant hepatitis B is high; 67% of affected infants die without liver transplantation [51]. Regarding older children or adolescents with fulminant hepatitis B, HBV infection occurs via a horizontal route (i.e., blood transfusion), which could potentially be prevented by infant vaccination or blood products screening [43].

Chronic HBV Infection

The natural course of chronic HBV infection, which is defined as persistence of HBsAg for more than 6 months, consists of three to four phases, according to the serum HBeAg and HBV DNA status.

Phase 1: Immune Tolerance Phase

Patients with chronic HBV infection have an initial immune tolerance state, which is characterized by the presence of HBeAg and high levels of HBV DNA due to rapid viral replication. The host is highly infectious, and an important source of horizontal infection in the family. During this phase, the host is usually asymptomatic and aminotransferase levels are usually normal, or mildly elevated. This phase is mostly seen in patients infected at birth or during early childhood. Infected children do not mount effective immune responses and exhibit immune tolerance, which leads to a high risk of chronicity in adulthood. Despite high levels of HBV DNA, liver damage in this phase is absent or minimal as a consequence of T cell immune tolerance to HBeAg and HBcAg [51]. Mechanisms underlying this immune tolerance are not well understood. During this phase, positivity of HBeAg and high HBV DNA levels in blood can persist for years after primary infection.

Phase 2: Inflammatory (Immune Active) Phase

When the host immune system becomes mature and begins to recognize HBV-related epitopes on hepatocytes, immune-mediated viral clearance and hepatocyte damage begin [52]. This phase, which lasts from several months to many years, is characterized by HBeAg positivity, high levels of HBV DNA, but now elevated serum aminotransferase levels, and active inflammation of the liver. In patients with perinatal or early childhood infection, transition from immune tolerance to immune clearance occurs mainly during the second or third decade of life [53]. Children in the HBe seroconversion stage mostly remain asymptomatic, or have mild non-specific symptoms such as general malaise, poor appetite, etc., making it difficult to detect the beginning of immune clearance. Serum ALT levels become elevated and fluctuate depending on the severity of liver damage during the virus–host interaction process. The peak levels of ALT often vary and are mostly <600 IU/mL. Active inflammation and hepatocyte damage are common histologic findings, but liver cirrhosis occurs uncommonly during childhood. Only 3.4% of 292 Italian HBsAg carrier children with elevated ALT were found to have liver cirrhosis at presentation [54].

The HBe seroconversion process, implying that the host loses the immune tolerance, varies in different individuals and is affected by age and maternal HBsAg status [55]. Some patients present with a flare of hepatitis followed by the disappearance of HBeAg and the presence of antibodies against HBeAg (anti-HBe); some have transient decreased HBV DNA levels without the clearance of HBeAg. In general, it takes around 2–7 years for the process of HBe seroconversion. The annual HBe seroconversion rate is less than 2% before the age of 3 years in a Taiwanese cohort; after 3 years of age, the annual HBe seroconversion rate gradually increased to about 5% [56].

Phase 3: Low Replication Phase (Inactive Carrier State)

After HBeAg seroconversion, most patients remain positive for anti-HBe antibodies and have gradual normalization of serum ALT levels. Patients in this phase are commonly referred to as "inactive HBsAg carriers." HBV DNA can only be detected in 1% of anti-HBe-positive children using the less sensitive hybridization method but can be persistently detected in sera, usually at less than 10^4 copies/mL, in the long term by assays that use the polymerase chain reaction (PCR). In an Italian study, 87% of 37 children after HBeAg seroconversion had detectable HBV DNA by PCR at 5-year follow-up and 58% had HBV DNA at 10-year follow-up [57]. Histologically minimal or mild hepatitis may be observed in children after HBeAg seroconversion.

Reactivation of HBV replication and a rise in ALT levels are not common in this phase in children; however, permanent liver damage and integration of the HBV genome may develop insidiously and gradually despite clearance of HBeAg. The subsequent development of liver cirrhosis or HCC is rarely observed but may happen during childhood [58]. In general, however, around 80% of childhood HCC occurs in children with anti-HBe antibodies [39, 59]. In an Italian long-term follow-up study for 29 years, the overall prognosis in horizontally infected children after HBeAg seroconversion showed that 2% of them progressed to HCC and 6% had HBeAg-negative hepatitis [60].

Phase 4: Reactivation Phase (HBeAg Negative Chronic Hepatitis B)

HBeAg seroconversion is generally considered as a good event indicating the cessation of liver inflammation and the beginning of an immune inactive status with low viral replication and minimal liver inflammation. However, HBeAg negative hepatitis is an important cause of liver injury after HBeAg seroconversion in adults. Subsequent reactivation of chronic hepatitis B occurs in up to one-third of inactive adult HBV carriers without reversion of HBeAg [61, 62]. This phase is characterized by the absence of HBeAg, the presence of anti-HBe antibodies, detectable HBV DNA levels ($<10^4$ copies/mL), serum ALT elevations, and histologically continuous necroinflammation of the liver. Most patients progress to this phase after a variable duration in the inactive carrier state, but some directly progress into this phase from immune clearance phase [63]. Selected HBV variants that cannot express HBeAg because of mutations in the precore or core regions of the HBV genome are thought to be the cause of HBeAg-negative chronic hepatitis [64].

The significance of HBeAg seroconversion occurring in childhood and young adulthood is clarified after a long-term follow-up study of 7–23.7 years [65]. In contrast to HBeAg seroconversion in adults, most children who underwent HBeAg seroconversion early had decreased viral loads, normal ALT levels, and uneventful courses after the HBeAg seroconversion. A prospective follow-up study of children with chronic hepatitis B showed that only 4.3% of 140 HBeAg seroconverters had re-elevated ALT after seroconversion [66].

Factors Affecting the Natural Course of Hepatitis B Virus Infection

Interactions between virus and the host may determine the natural course of HBV infection in an individual. Maternal factors may also affect the disease process in children who acquire HBV infection perinatally.

Maternal Factors

Children with HBeAg-positive mothers have higher rates of chronic infection (around 90%) after perinatal HBV transmission and lower rates of HBe seroconversion during long-term follow-up than those with HBeAg-negative mothers. This might be due to exposure to transplacental maternal HBeAg in utero since it has been demonstrated that there is absence of T cell response to HBcAg in children of HBeAg-positive mothers [51]. In contrast, infants of HBeAg-negative mothers are prone to acute hepatitis B with recovery, or fulminant hepatitis B with a high mortality rate of approximately 67% [50].

Viral Factors

HBV genotype and variants also play a role. In one study, children with genotype C had late HBeAg seroconversion compared to that in those with genotype B during a 15-year follow-up period [67]. The HBV precore stop codon mutation [68], basal core promoter mutation [69], and core gene deletion mutation [70] may influence HBe seroconversion in children. An analysis of long-term followed 80 HBV-infected children revealed an increased proportion of the precore stop codon mutant of G to A mutation at nucleotide 1896 position after HBeAg seroconversion (50%), increased from 10% at the early HBeAg-positive stage [68]. An age-matched case–control longitudinal study showed that precore 1896 mutant accounts for half of childhood HBeAg seroconversion, and mutations of core promoter at nucleotide position 1752, 1755, and 1799 also have significant correlation with HBeAg seroconversion, whereas core promoter 1762/1764 mutations play a minimal role in HBeAg seroconversion in children [69].

Core gene mutations at codons 74, 87, and 159 are frequently seen in HBV-infected children with HCC, whereas codons 21, 147, and 65 are mostly seen in children with chronic HBV infection without HCC [71]. A long-term follow-up study demonstrated that core gene deletion mutants appeared in 4.9% of 365 children with chronic hepatitis B and mostly signified HBeAg seroconversion within 1 year [70]. Mutations of the human leukocyte antigen-A2-restricted T-cell epitope (TCE) on the HBsAg region were demonstrated to be positively associated with early HBeAg seroconversion and higher ALT levels in children with chronic hepatitis B [72]. Children who have relatively lower HBV DNA levels (<1,000 pg/mL, equivalent to 5×10^7 IU/mL) have a higher rate of undergoing HBeAg seroconversion during the subsequent 1–3 years than those with higher levels of viremia [56].

Host Factors

Children who have elevated ALT of >100 IU/mL often (66.7%, 16/24 cases) undergo HBeAg seroconversion during the subsequent 1–3 years, in comparison with 17.6% (27/153) in those with <100 IU/mL [56]. Cytokines also play roles in directly inhibiting viral replication and indirectly determining the patterns of host immune response [73]. Higher levels of serum interleukin (IL)-12 (>45 pg/mL) and IL-10 (>70 pg/mL) have been associated with early spontaneous HBeAg seroconversion in children. Variations in host cytokine genes may influence HBeAg seroconversion individually. The IL-10-1082 G/G and IL-12 beta −10993 C/G genotypes also predict early spontaneous HBeAg seroconversion [74]. In men, earlier-onset puberty, which refers to serum testosterone levels >2.5 ng/mL at 15 years of age, and increased enzyme activity of steroid 5α-reductase type II (SRD5A2) are associated with earlier spontaneous HBeAg seroconversion [75]. Nevertheless, additional determinant host factors still need to be examined.

Conclusions

Global control and elimination of hepatitis B virus infection remain an important and challenging task. The epidemiology, natural history, and treatment concerns are significantly different between children and adults with HBV infection. Decisions on when and how to treat are still difficult in asymptomatic children, and prevention should always be the preferred strategy. Any comprehensive strategy against HBV infection should include prevention of perinatal transmission, vaccination in considerable populations, and interruption of nosocomial transmission. The effects of global prevention of new infections will be apparent in decades.

References

1. Ganem D, Prince AM. Hepatitis B virus infection natural history and clinical consequences. N Engl J Med. 2004;350:1118–1129.
2. Kane MA. Global status of hepatitis B immunization. Lancet. 1996;348:696.
3. Margolis HS. Fact sheets for candidate diseases for elimination or eradication. Hepatitis B virus infection. Bull World Health Organ. 1998;76:152–153.

4. Harpaz R, McMahon BJ, Margolis HS, et al. Elimination of new chronic hepatitis B infections: results of the Alaska immunization program. J Infect Dis. 2000;181:413–418.
5. Ni YH, Huang LM, Chang MH, et al. Two decades of universal hepatitis B vaccination in Taiwan: impact and implication for future strategies. Gastroenterology. 2007;132:1287–1293.
6. Montesano R. Hepatitis B immunization and hepatocellular carcinoma: the Gambia Hepatitis Intervention Study. J Med Virol. 2002;67:444–446.
7. Viviani S, Jack A, Hall AJ, et al. Hepatitis B vaccination in infancy in The Gambia: protection against carriage at 9 years of age. Vaccine. 1999;17:2946–2950.
8. Da Villa G, Sepe A. Immunization programme against hepatitis B virus infection in Italy: cost-effectiveness. Vaccine. 1999;17:1734–1738.
9. Salleras L, Domínguez A, Bruguera M, et al. Declining prevalence of hepatitis B virus infection in Catalonia (Spain) 12 years after the introduction of universal vaccination. Vaccine. 2007;25:8726–8731.
10. Sun Z, Ming L, Zhu X, Lu J. Prevention and control of hepatitis B in China. J Med Virol. 2002;67:447–450.
11. Liang X, Bi S, Yang W, et al. Epidemiological serosurvey of hepatitis B in China-declining HBV prevalence due to hepatitis B vaccination. Vaccine. 2009;27:6550–6557.
12. Al-Faleh FZ, Al-Jeffri M, Ramia S, et al. Seroepidemiology of hepatitis B virus infection in Saudi children 8 years after a mass hepatitis B vaccination programme. J Infect. 1999;38:167–170.
13. Ruff TA, Gertig DM, Otto BF, et al. Lombok Hepatitis B Model Immunization Project: toward universal infant hepatitis B immunization in Indonesia. J Infect Dis. 1995;171:290–296.
14. Chunsuttiwat S, Biggs BA, Maynard J, et al. Integration of hepatitis B vaccination into the expanded programme on immunization in Chonburi and Chiangmai provinces, Thailand. Vaccine. 1997;15:769–774.
15. McQuillan GM, Coleman PJ, Kruszon-Moran D, et al. Prevalence of hepatitis B virus infection in the United States: the National Health and Nutrition Examination Surveys, 1976 through 1994. Am J Public Health. 1999;89:14–18.
16. Centers for Disease Control and Prevention. Acute hepatitis B among children and adolescents: United States, 1990–2002. MMWR Morb Mortal Wkly Rep. 2004;53:1015–1018.
17. Zhang J, Zou S, Giulivi A. Epidemiology of hepatitis B in Canada. Can J Infect Dis. 2001;12:345–350.
18. Alter MJ. Protecting future generations through immunization against hepatitis B. Ann Intern Med. 2001;135:835–836.
19. Custer B, Sullivan SD, Hazlet TK, et al. Global epidemiology of hepatitis B virus. J Clin Gastroenterol. 2004;38:S158–S168.
20. Goudeau A. Epidemiology and eradication strategy for hepatitis B in Europe: the European Regional Study Group. Vaccine. 1990;8:113–116.
21. Van Damme P, Vorsters A. Hepatitis B control in Europe by universal vaccination programmes: the situation in 2001. J Med Virol. 2002;67:433–439.
22. Stroffolini T, Mele A, Tosti ME, et al. The impact of the hepatitis B mass immunisation campaign on the incidence and risk factors of acute hepatitis B in Italy. J Hepatol. 2000; 33:980–985.
23. Merican I, Guan R, Amarapuka D, et al. Chronic hepatitis B virus infection in Asian countries. J Gastroenterol Hepatol. 2000;15:1356–1361.
24. Hsu HY, Chang MH, Chen DS, Lee CY, Sung JL. Baseline seroepidemiology of hepatitis B virus infection in children in Taipei, 1984: a study just before mass hepatitis B vaccination program in Taiwan. J Med Virol. 1986;18:301–307.
25. Kiire CF. Hepatitis B infection in sub-Saharan Africa: the African Regional Study Group. Vaccine. 1990;8:107–112.
26. André F. Hepatitis B epidemiology in Asia, the Middle East and Africa. Vaccine. 2000; 18:S20–S22.
27. Edmunds WJ, Medley GF, Nokes DJ. The transmission dynamics and control of hepatitis B virus in The Gambia. Stat Med. 1996;15:2215–2233.

28. Edmunds WJ, Medley GF, Nokes DJ, et al. Epidemiologic patterns of hepatitis B virus (HBV) in highly endemic areas. Epidemiol Infect. 1996;117:313–325.
29. Kiire CF. The epidemiology and prophylaxis of hepatitis B in sub-Saharan Africa: a view from tropical and subtropical Africa. Gut. 1996;38:S5–S12.
30. Hsu HM, Chen DS, Chuang CH, et al. Efficacy of a mass hepatitis B vaccination program in Taiwan. Studies on 3464 infants of hepatitis B surface antigen-carrier mothers. JAMA. 1988;260:2231–2235.
31. Yang YJ, Liu CC, Chen TJ, et al. Role of hepatitis B immunoglobulin in infants born to hepatitis B e antigen-negative carrier mothers in Taiwan. Pediatr Infect Dis J. 2003;22:584–588.
32. Beasley RP, Hwang LY, Lin CC, et al. Incidence of hepatitis B virus infections in preschool children in Taiwan. J Infect Dis. 1982;146:198–204.
33. Beasley RP, Hwang LY, Lin CC, Ko YC, Twu SJ. Incidence of hepatitis among students at a university in Taiwan. Am J Epidemiol. 1983;117:213–222.
34. McMahon BJ, Alward WL, Hall DB, et al. Acute hepatitis B virus infection: relation of age to the clinical expression of disease and subsequent development of the carrier state. J Infect Dis. 1985;151:599–603.
35. Stevens CE, Beasley RP, Tsui J, Lee WC. Vertical transmission of hepatitis B antigen in Taiwan. N Engl J Med. 1975;292:771–774.
36. Lee SD, Tsai YT, Wu TC, et al. Role of caesarean section in prevention of mother–infant transmission of hepatitis B virus. Lancet. 1988;2:833–834.
37. Wang J, Zhu Q, Zhang X. Effect of delivery mode on maternal–infant transmission of hepatitis B virus by immunoprophylaxis. Chin Med J. 2002;115:1510–1512.
38. Chang MH. Hepatitis B virus infection. Semin Fetal Neonatal Med. 2007;12:160–167.
39. Chang MH, Chen CJ, Lai MS, et al. Universal hepatitis B vaccination in Taiwan and the incidence of hepatocellular carcinoma in children. N Engl J Med. 1997;336:1855–1859.
40. Chang MH, Shau WY, Chen CJ, et al. Hepatitis B vaccination and hepatocellular carcinoma rates in boys and girls. JAMA. 2000;284:3040–3042.
41. Chang MH, Chen TH, Hsu HM, et al. Prevention of hepatocellular carcinoma by universal vaccination against hepatitis B virus: the effect and problems. Clin Cancer Res. 2005; 11:7953–7957.
42. Chang MH, You SL, Chen CJ, et al. Decreased incidence of hepatocellular carcinoma in hepatitis B vaccinees: a 20-year follow-up study. J Natl Cancer Inst. 2009;101:1348–1355.
43. Chen HL, Chang CJ, Kong MS, et al. Pediatric fulminant hepatic failure in endemic areas of hepatitis B infection: 15 years after universal hepatitis B vaccination. Hepatology. 2004;39:58–63.
44. Chien YC, Jan CF, Kuo HS, Chen CJ. Nationwide hepatitis B vaccination program in Taiwan: effectiveness in the 20 years after it was launched. Epidemiol Rev. 2006;28:126–135.
45. Yotsuyanagi H, Yasuda K, Iino S, et al. Persistent viremia after recovery from self-limited acute hepatitis B. Hepatology. 1998;27:1377–1382.
46. Blanpain C, Knoop C, Delforge ML, et al. Reactivation of hepatitis B after transplantation in patients with pre-existing anti-hepatitis B surface antigen antibodies: report on three cases and review of the literature. Transplantation. 1998;66:883–886.
47. Bhaduri BR, Mieli-Vergani G. Fulminant hepatic failure: pediatric aspects. Semin Liver Dis. 1996;16:349–355.
48. Bernuau J, Rueff B, Benhamou JP. Fulminant and subfulminant liver failure: definitions and causes. Semin Liver Dis. 1986;6:97–106.
49. Lee WS, McKiernan P, Kelly DA. Etiology, outcome and prognostic indicators of childhood fulminant hepatic failure in the United Kingdom. J Pediatr Gastroenterol Nutr. 2005; 40:575–581.
50. Chang MH, Lee CY, Chen DS, Hsu HC, Lai MY. Fulminant hepatitis in children in Taiwan: the important role of hepatitis B virus. J Pediatr. 1987;111:34–39.
51. Hsu HY, Chang MH, Hsieh KH, et al. Cellular immune response to HBeAg in mother-to-infant transmission of hepatitis B virus. Hepatology. 1992;15:770–776.

52. Chu CM, Liaw YF. Intrahepatic distribution of hepatitis B surface and core antigens in chronic hepatitis B virus infection: hepatocyte with cytoplasmic/membranous hepatitis B core antigen as a possible target for immune hepatocytolysis. Gastroenterology. 1987;92:220–225.
53. Liaw YF, Tai DI, Chu CM, Pao CC, Chen TJ. Acute exacerbation in chronic type B hepatitis: comparison between HBeAg and antibody-positive patients. Hepatology. 1987;7:20–23.
54. Bortolotti F, Cadrobbi P, Crivellaro C, et al. Long-term outcome of chronic type B hepatitis in patients who acquire hepatitis B virus in infection in childhood. Gastroenterology. 1990;99:805–810.
55. Chang MH, Sung JL, Lee CY, Chen JS, Hsu HY, Lee PI, et al. Factors affecting clearance of hepatitis B e antigen in hepatitis B surface antigen carrier children. J Pediatr. 1989;115: 385–390.
56. Lee PI, Chang MH, Lee CY et al. Changes of serum hepatitis B virus DNA and aminotransferase levels during the course of chronic hepatitis B virus infection in children. Hepatology. 1990;12:657–660.
57. Bortolotti F, Wirth S, Crivellaro C, Alberti A, Martine U, de Moliner L. Long-term persistence of hepatitis B virus DNA in the serum of children with chronic hepatitis B after hepatitis B e antigen to antibody seroconversion. J Pediatr Gastroenterol Nutr. 1996;22:270–274.
58. Bortolotti F, Calzia R, Cadrobbi P, Crivellaro C, Alberti A, Marazzi MG. Long-term evolution of chronic hepatitis B in children with antibody to hepatitis B e antigen. J Pediatr. 1990;116:552–555.
59. Chang MH, Chen PJ, Chen JY, et al. Hepatitis B virus integration in hepatitis B virus-related hepatocellular carcinoma in childhood. Hepatology. 1991;13:316–320.
60. Bortolotti F, Cuido M, Bartolacci S, et al. Chronic hepatitis B in children after e antigen seroclearance: final report of a 29-year longitudinal study. Hepatology. 2006;43:556–562.
61. Sung JJ, Chan HL, Wong ML, et al. Relationship of clinical and virological factors with hepatitis activity in hepatitis B e antigen-negative chronic hepatitis B virus-infected patients. J Viral Hepat. 2002;9:229–234.
62. Funk ML, Rosenberg DM, Lok AS. World-wide epidemiology of HBeAg-negative chronic hepatitis B and associated precore and core promoter variants. J Viral Hepat. 2002;9:52–61.
63. Hsu YS, Chien RN, Yeh CT, et al. Long-term outcome after spontaneous HBeAg seroconversion in patients with chronic hepatitis B. Hepatology. 2002;35:1522–1527.
64. Hadziyannis SJ, Vassilopoulos D. Hepatitis B e antigen-negative chronic hepatitis B. Hepatology. 2001;34:617–624.
65. Ni YH, Chang MH, Chen PJ, Tsai KS, Hsu HY, Chen HL, Tsuei DJ, Chen DS. Viremia profiles in children with chronic hepatitis B virus infection and spontaneous e antigen seroconversion. Gastroenterology. 2007;132:2340–2345.
66. Chang MH, Hsu HY, Hsu HC, Ni YH, Chen JS, Chen DS. The significance of spontaneous hepatitis B e antigen seroconversion in childhood: with special emphasis on the clearance of hepatitis B e antigen before 3 years of age. Hepatology. 1995;22:1387–1392.
67. Ni YH, Chang MH, Wang KJ, et al. Clinical relevance of hepatitis B virus genotype in children with chronic infection and hepatocellular carcinoma. Gastroenterology. 2004;127: 1733–1738.
68. Chang MH, Hsu HY, Ni YH, et al. Precore stop codon mutant in chronic hepatitis B virus infection in children: its relation to hepatitis B e seroconversion and maternal hepatitis B surface antigen. J Hepatol. 1998;28:915–922.
69. Ni YH, Chang MH, Hsu HY, Tsuei DJ. Longitudinal study on mutation profiles of core promoter and precore regions of the hepatitis B virus genome in children. Pediatr Res. 2004;56: 396–399.
70. Ni YH, Chang MH, Hsu HY, Chen HL. Long-term follow-up study of core gene deletion mutants in children with chronic hepatitis B virus infection. Hepatology. 2000;32:124–128.
71. Ni YH, Chang MH, Hsu HY, Tsuei DJ. Different hepatitis B virus core gene mutations in children with chronic infection and hepatocellular carcinoma. Gut. 2003;52:122–125.
72. Ni YH, Chang MH, Hsu HY, et al. Mutations of T-cell epitopes in the hepatitis B virus surface gene in children with chronic infection and hepatocellular carcinoma. Am J Gastroenterol. 2008;103:1004–1009.

73. Koziel MJ. Cytokines in viral hepatitis. Semin Liver Dis. 1999;19:157–169.
74. Wu JF, Wu TC, Chen CH, et al. Serum levels of interleukin-10 and interleukin-12 predict early, spontaneous hepatitis B virus e antigen seroconversion. Gastroenterology. 2010;138: 165–172.
75. Wu JF, Tsai WY, Hsu HY, et al. Effect of puberty onset on spontaneous hepatitis B virus e antigen seroconversion in men. Gastroenterology. 2010;138:942–948.

Treatment of Chronic Hepatitis B in Children

Annemarie Broderick

Key Concepts

- Awareness of the natural history of chronic hepatitis B infection in children is central to any decisions regarding treatment.
- A child with chronic HBV infection should have serological markers of HBV infection (HBsAg, HBeAg, and/or HBV DNA) on two occasions at least 6 months apart to be considered for treatment.
- A liver biopsy may be helpful before starting treatment.
- Therapeutic goals include long-term suppression of HBV replication, cessation of liver injury, and reduction of risk for cirrhosis and hepatocellular carcinoma.
- Currently, six agents in two classes (interferons and nucleot(s)ide analogs) are available for treatment of chronic HBV infection but only interferon-alfa and lamivudine are licensed in USA for children less than 12 years of age.
- There is limited information regarding the use of other nucleot(s)ide analogs in children, although studies are ongoing.
- Co-infections with hepatitis C or human immunodeficiency virus require special approaches to treatment of chronic HBV infection.
- Given concerns about the long-term natural history, the limited therapeutic options, and the serious risk of resistance to antiviral agents, an optimal treatment regimen for children with chronic hepatitis B infection has not yet been developed, and clinicians should use these agents prudently.

Keywords Interferon-α • Lamivudine • Adefovir dipivoxil • Nucleoside • Nucleotide • Management • Co-infection • Hepatitis C • HIV

A. Broderick (✉)
School of Medicine and Medical Science, University College Dublin, Dublin 4, Ireland
e-mail: annemarie.broderick@ucd.ie

M.M. Jonas (ed.), *Viral Hepatitis in Children: Unique Features and Opportunities*, Clinical Gastroenterology, DOI 10.1007/978-1-60761-373-2_3,

Introduction

In the last two decades, drug treatment options for chronic hepatitis B virus (HBV) infection have increased from just one agent to six. These include five oral nucleos(t)ide analogs as well as interferon (IFN)-α. This progress has brought greater complexity to the therapy decision-making process. Treatment decisions now involve patient selection, timing, and determination of the best agent. This chapter deals with these clinical dilemmas in childhood where there are additional confounders, such as the natural history of HBV infection in youngsters and the ramifications for growth, development, and a long life expectancy.

Acute Hepatitis B

Infants who acquire HBV infection perinatally usually have no symptoms or signs and go on to develop chronic HBV infections. Older children may develop clinical and biochemical signs of acute hepatitis at the time of infection and in exceptional circumstances, treatment may be considered. The current American Association for the Study of Liver Diseases (AASLD) guideline recommends treatment for patients with acute or fulminant liver failure due to HBV, or for those with prolonged, severe acute hepatitis B [1, 2]. These recommendations are based on two studies in adults. In the first, lamivudine was administered to 17 patients with fulminant HBV in a German center. Of these, 14 recovered without liver transplantation, two required transplants, and one died from cerebral herniation. An additional 20 patients from five other centers were also included in the report, of which 15 survived without transplantation [3]. In a randomized control trial of 71 adult patients (31 lamivudine, 40 placebo) reported from India, lamivudine decreased HBV DNA level more than placebo but there was no difference in clinical outcome [4]. There are no data regarding treatment of acute HBV in children.

Chronic Hepatitis B

The ideal goals of therapy of chronic hepatitis B are eradication of HBV, improvement of liver disease, and prevention of hepatocellular carcinoma (HCC). Endpoints of treatment can be virological, such as cessation of viral replication as indicated by loss of hepatitis B e antigen (HBeAg) or HBV DNA, or clearance of hepatitis B surface antigen (HBsAg) from serum; histological, i.e., normalization of liver histopathology; and biochemical, with normalization of aminotransferase values. To date, no single agent fulfills all of these goals in either adults or children. For practical purposes, suppression of HBV viral load to levels undetectable by sensitive techniques such as polymerase chain reaction (PCR) rather than complete eradication may be more realistic, as eradication is difficult to achieve.

Treatment of children is further complicated by differences in immune tolerance, immune clearance, and rate of progression of liver disease in children compared to that in adults. Therefore, studies of treatments for chronic HBV in adults cannot be extrapolated directly to children.

A child being considered for treatment must have serological evidence of HBV infection, i.e., be HBsAg positive for at least 6 months, as well as evidence of active HBV replication, i.e., either be HBeAg positive or have measurable levels of HBV DNA in serum. Children with very low HBV DNA levels may be in the process of spontaneous seroconversion; therefore, an expectant policy may be prudent. These factors are summarized in Table 1. Children with consistent elevation of alanine aminotransferase (ALT) to at least twice the upper limit of normal (ULN) are most likely to benefit from treatment. A liver biopsy should be obtained before the start of therapy to stage the disease and to rule out other disease processes (Table 2).

Defining study outcomes in a clinically meaningful way in chronic hepatitis B is difficult, since the disease may take decades to progress, and yet studies, by their nature, cover a pre-defined and usually short period of time. The time after cessation of therapy (6 or 12 months) has been used to define a sustained response. A number of practical endpoints are used; virological, histological, biochemical, and clinical, as summarized in Table 3. Endpoints are discussed in general below and specifically for each treatment agent.

Table 1 Factors favoring treatment of chronic HBV infection during childhood

Persistent elevation of ALT greater than two times ULN and persistent elevation of HBV DNA>20,000 IU/ml (4 log IU/ml)
Moderate/severe inflammation or significant fibrosis on liver biopsy
Risk factors or serological evidence of other types of liver disease
Family history of HBV-associated HCC
Co-infection with HIV
Requirement for immunosuppression or chemotherapy

Table 2 When to consider liver biopsy in children with chronic HBV

Persistent elevation of ALT and elevation of HBV DNA≥20,000 IU/mL
Abnormal imaging suggestive of cirrhosis
To evaluate for other etiologies of liver disease, such as non-alcoholic fatty liver in obese children or adolescents

Table 3 Target outcomes in treatment of chronic HBV in children

Category	Outcome
Virological	Conversion from HBeAg to anti-HBe
	Loss of HBV DNA from serum
	Conversion from HBsAg to anti-HBs
Clinical	Prevention of chronic liver disease
	Reduction in life-time risk of hepatocellular carcinoma
Biochemical	Normalization of ALT
Histopathological	Decrease in inflammatory activity on liver biopsy

Virological Responses

The virological responses used to define successful treatment differ among studies and it is therefore important to evaluate fully the criteria used before comparing outcomes. Traditional virological endpoints have been seroconversion from HBeAg to anti-HBe and complete suppression of HBV DNA. Assessing outcomes has become more complex for a number of reasons. The emergence of HBeAg-negative chronic HBV infection has limited the use of HBeAg as a marker, and although this form of infection is unusual in children, it is becoming increasingly reported. Quantifying HBV DNA is not straightforward as a number of different tests and methods are used to measure the viral load. The range of each assay is different, as are the units of reporting. The World Health Organization (WHO) has created a standardized unit of measurement, the international unit (IU/mL), and this unit is recommended for use in clinical trials [5]. Finally, the increasing use of nucleoside or nucleotide analogs will change outcome measures as response not only needs to be sustained but also maintained long term [6]. Loss of HBsAg is seldom used as an outcome measure as it is an infrequent occurrence, but it is usually reported if it occurs.

Clinical Responses

Most children with chronic HBV infection report no symptoms; therefore, the absence of symptoms is not usually included as treatment outcome. IFN may impair quality of life dramatically due to treatment-related side effects. Reassuringly, quality of life recovers to pre-IFN levels within 3 months of completion of treatment [7] and side effects typically resolve completely. Chronic HBV infection is a risk factor for the development of HCC, but as this is uncommon in childhood, epidemiological studies rather than treatment series yield more useful information. Since 1984, all newborns in Taiwan have been vaccinated against HBV. After approximately 10 years of universal vaccination, a significant decrease in the incidence of HCC in children aged 6–14 years was reported, from 0.70 per 100,000 children (97 children) between 1981 and 1986 to 0.36 per 100,000 (49 children) between 1990 and 1994 [8]. Very long-term studies will be required to study whether the incidence will be reduced in the sixth decade of life, the peak age for HCC in perinatally infected individuals.

Biochemical Responses

Children with aminotransferase elevation to at least twice the ULN are more likely to respond to treatment with IFN-α or lamivudine. Serum ALT is a surrogate marker of hepatic inflammation and commonly normalizes during treatment. However, it should be used in combination with other endpoints as it has limited predictive value. Measurement of ALT is useful, however, in monitoring treatment-associated hepatitis flares [9].

Histopathological Responses

In HBV infection, a liver biopsy is used to quantify the severity of changes, to rule out other causes of liver disease, and occasionally to assess changes after treatment. The histopathological findings of chronic HBV infection are portal tract inflammation, interface hepatitis, and fibrosis, which may progress to architectural distortion of lobules and eventual cirrhosis [10]. Histopathological staging and grading systems are used to allow standardization and meaningful comparisons in several types of chronic hepatitis. One such system is the Knodell–Ishak score which evaluates four histopathological features – each scored using specific criteria [11]. This system has proved reproducible, and is now is in common use as the modified histological activity index (HAI). Other scoring methods are the Batts–Ludwig system [12] and METAVIR system [13]. These systematic classifications are useful in estimating progression of disease and response to therapy, and for comparing outcomes in therapeutic trials. A study from Poland demonstrated that these scores were useful in comparing liver biopsies in children before and after IFN-α treatment for chronic hepatitis B, and that inflammatory but not fibrosis scores improved after treatment [14]. However, another study demonstrated inter-observer variability in grading and staging of pediatric liver biopsy specimens [15]. Clinicians must be aware of these limitations of liver biopsies [15].

Serum markers of hepatic fibrosis, such as apolipoprotein A-1, haptoglobin, and A-2 macroglobulin, have been investigated in children. They present many theoretical advantages for non-invasive monitoring of patients, but no single marker has yet been proven useful in children with chronic HBV infection [16].

Medications

Medications used to treat chronic HBV infection, and occasionally acute HBV infection, can be divided into two groups: the interferon family, and oral nucleoside and nucleotide agents.

Interferon

The interferons are a family of cytokines with immunomodulatory, antiproliferative, and direct antiviral actions. There are three types: α, β, and γ. IFN-α has been the primary form used for chronic HBV infection and induces the display of HLA class I molecules on hepatocyte membranes, which in turn promotes lysis by $CD8^+$ cytotoxic lymphocytes. At the same time, it directly inhibits viral protein synthesis [17]. IFN-α was first reported as a successful treatment for chronic HBV in 1976 [18] and recombinant IFN-α_{2b} was approved by the US Food and Drug Administration for chronic HBV in 1992 for adults and in 1998 for children. IFN-α is currently available as IFN-α_{2a}, IFN-α_{2b}, and lymphoblastoid IFN-α. These are summarized in Table 4. Only IFN-α_{2b} has been licensed in USA for use in children. Peginterferon α_{2a}, interferon linked to polyethylene glycol to slow absorption and is thus appropriate for weekly use, has not yet been studied or licensed for use in children with chronic HBV.

Children with evidence of active immunological responses to HBV (immune active phase), i.e., low to moderate levels of HBV DNA and ALT values greater than twice the ULN, are more likely to respond to therapy with IFN-α [19]. If only children with elevated aminotransferases are selected for treatment with IFN-α, then children younger than 13 years of age with intermediate HBV DNA levels are most likely to have a good response, regardless of ethnicity [20]. In a large multinational, randomized control trial of IFN-α_{2b}, no differences were found in loss of HBeAg between children born in Asian countries (22%) and those from Europe and North America (26%) if aminotransferase values were elevated [20]. In other studies, ethnic differences were more pronounced. IFN-α treatment led to loss of HBV DNA or HBeAg seroconversion in 20–58% of European compared with 8–17% of control children [21], but in a study from Asia only 3–17% cleared HBV DNA or had HBeAg seroconversion [22]. These children may well have been in the immune-tolerant phase of HBV infection.

Long-term (1.1–11.5 years) follow-up of adult responders to IFN-α showed a significantly reduced incidence of HCC compared with either treated nonresponders or control patients [23]. The long-term outlook for treated children is not yet clear. In a Turkish study, none of 23 treatment non-responders developed cirrhosis or HCC, but mean follow-up was only 4.5 years [24]. A second study compared long-term (5.6 ± 3.1 years) outcome in two groups of 37 children, one group treated with IFN-α_{2b} and a group of children matched for age, sex, and baseline ALT level who received no treatment. At follow-up, the rates of HBeAg and HBsAg loss were 54.1% (20/37) and 8.1% (3/37) in treated children compared to 35.1% (13/37) and 2.7% (1/37), respectively, in untreated children (NS). Treated children with ALT levels elevated more than two times ULN had higher rates of HBeAg seroconversion at follow-up compared to children with elevated ALT who were not treated [25]. A study from Sweden demonstrated that lower (HBV DNA < 8.2 log IU/ml) pretreatment HBV DNA levels were associated with sustained virological response [26].

In children and young adults in Taiwan, no long-term advantage of IFN-α therapy was observed. A group of 42 children were followed for between 6.5 and 12.5 years; 21 received no treatment and 21 were treated with IFN alone (17) or with IFN and prednisolone (4). All children treated in this trial were HBeAg and HBsAg positive with ALT values greater than twice ULN on two occasions at least

Table 4 Interferon for chronic HBV in children: types, doses, and frequency of administration

Drug	Dose	Frequency	References	Approved by FDA for use in children with chronic hepatitis B
Interferon α-2b (Intron A® Schering Plough Corporation)	3 $MU/m^2/day$	Three times a week × 24 weeks	[27]	Yes
	3 $MU/m^2/day$ (week 1)	Week 1 only	[20]	
	6 $MU/m^2/day$	Three times a week × 16–24 weeks	[20]	
	5 $MU/m^2/day$ or 10 $MU/m^2/day$	Three times a week × 24 weeks	[99]	
Interferon α-2a (Roferon-A®, Hoffmann-LaRoche)	3 $MU/m^2/day$ or 7.5 $MU/m^2/day$	Three times a week × 24 weeks	[100]	No
Human lymphoblastoid interferon α	5 $MU/m^2/day$ (week 1), then up to 10 $MU/m^2/day$	Three times a week × 12 weeks	[101]	No

6 months apart before enrollment. Those (4/5) with a sustained virological response 12 months after the end of treatment had lower baseline HBV DNA levels ($\leq 2 \times 10^8$ copies/ml) than those (12/13) who did not respond to treatment (HBV DNA levels $\geq 2 \times 10^8$ copies/ml) [27]. Higher success rates in children with lower HBV DNA values were also noted in an open prospective Swedish study [26]. A total of 27 children were treated and all displayed evidence of being in the immune active stage of chronic HBV infection. Lower pretreatment HBV DNA levels appear to be a predictor of response. The authors caution that the small numbers in this trial may explain the lack of association between high pretreatment ALT levels and response noted in previous trials.

Two meta-analyses of treatment of chronic HBV in children with IFN-α have been conducted [19, 28]. Each report concludes that treatment leads to a higher rate of HBeAg seroconversion than would occur spontaneously. Randomized control trials may be analyzed for "number to treat" (i.e., the number of children requiring treatment in order to have a therapeutic response in one patient). If only children with ALT values twice normal are considered, 2.5 children would need to be treated for one to clear HBV DNA. However, if all infected children are treated, then 7.1 children would require therapy to clear HBV DNA from one child [19]. Since approximately two-thirds of children treated with IFN-α show no sustained response to therapy, more effective and better-tolerated treatments are required.

A study in adults reported a greater benefit to treatment with IFN. A single-center study from the Netherlands of 165 patients with chronic HBV infection treated with IFN-α and with a median follow-up of 8.8 years (range 0.3–24 years) reported significantly improved survival rates (relative risk of death, 0.28) and reduced incidence of HCC (RR, 0.08) in responders (54/165 or 33%) [29]. This discrepancy may be due to study design: the adult study compared outcomes in responders to those in non-responders, while the pediatric study [27] compared all treated children (responders and non-responders) to those who received no treatment.

Polish investigators reported histological outcomes in 93 children, average age 7.1 years, with chronic HBV treated with IFN-α for 20 weeks. Liver biopsies were obtained before treatment and 12 months after the end of the treatment, and graded for fibrosis and inflammation using three different scoring systems. A total of 35 children underwent HBeAg seroconversion and 58 did not respond. Liver fibrosis did not improve regardless of response, but inflammatory activity was decreased after treatment in both groups [15].

Higher doses of IFN-α (10 megaunits)/m^2) are not associated with higher response rates, although treatment for 6 months seems to improve outcome compared to shorter courses [21]. In the multinational, randomized, controlled trial referenced previously, children received 6 megaunits(MU)/m^2 of IFN-α_{2b} three times a week for 6 months. However, the dose of IFN-α_{2b} had to be reduced in 23% of children because of bone marrow suppression or fever. Serum HBeAg and HBV DNA became negative in 26% of treated children and 11% of controls. In children who responded to therapy, liver histology improved, and serum aminotransferase values normalized [30]. Prednisone priming (i.e., a course of steroids immediately before IFN-α treatment) has been proposed to induce an acute exacerbation of hepatitis B, thereby rendering the patient more susceptible to IFN. However, a dual-center, double-blind, randomized trial of lymphoblastoid IFN-α with or without steroid pretreatment showed no improvement in HBeAg-to-HBeAb seroconversion rate over that of IFN-α alone [31], and this regimen is no longer used.

Side effects of IFN-α include a transient influenza-like syndrome (fever, myalgia, headache, arthralgia, and anorexia) that occurs in virtually all patients at the start of therapy. Bone marrow suppression, especially neutropenia, is common, seen in 39% of children in one series [7]. Changes in personality, irritability, and temper tantrums are reported more frequently in children than in adults [7, 20]. These problems resolve once treatment is withdrawn. Epistaxis not associated with thrombocytopenia or prolonged prothrombin time, febrile seizures, and marked elevation of aminotransferases have been reported. There is a report of death of a 5-year-old girl with chronic hepatitis B infection within hours of administration of the first dose of IFN-α_{2a} which may have been related to a hypersensitivity reaction [32]. Quality of life is impaired in children during IFN therapy compared with pretreatment because of medication side effects and fear of injections. However, within 3 months of cessation of treatment, these effects are reversed [7]. Therapy in children is seldom discontinued because of side effects or inability to administer the medication.

HBV Polymerase Inhibitors

This class of agents includes the nucleoside and nucleotide analogs that inhibit viral replication by HBV polymerase by incorporation into viral DNA, leading to termination. These agents suppress rather than eradicate HBV. They are administered orally and are generally well tolerated [33], making them an attractive class of agents. This class has proliferated in the last few years and there are now five agents available for use in adults. These are compared in Table 5. These drugs share a potentially serious class effect, weak inhibition of mitochondrial DNA polymerase gamma, which could lead to mitochondrial loss or dysfunction. Fortunately, this effect is rare in the five nucleos(t)ide agents approved for HBV infection but could manifest as lactic acidosis, hepatic steatosis, myopathy, neuropathy, and pancreatitis [34]. Patients and physicians need to be alert to these potential effects. Some of these drugs have been used in combination, with no apparent increase in the frequency of adverse events.

The first of this group to be licensed for treatment of chronic HBV was lamivudine (2′,3′-dideoxycytosine), also known as 3TC, an oral nucleoside analog. It is triphosphorylated intracellularly to an active intermediate that is incorporated into the growing DNA chain, thereby terminating the chain and inhibiting viral replication. Two large, randomized, controlled studies of lamivudine as initial treatment for chronic HBV infection in adults demonstrated serological, biochemical, and histological evidence of benefit [35, 36].

Table 5 Nucleoside/nucleotide analogs used for chronic hepatitis B

	Mechanism of action	Trials in children	Approved by FDA for use in children with chronic HBV infection	Trials in adults	HBV DNA viral load suppression	Resistance	Safety profile
Lamivudine	Inhibits reverse transcriptase (H Thomas et al. J Hepatol 2003 S93–98)	Yes [39]	Yes	Yes [36]	Yes [36, 39]	Frequent 30% by 1 year 70% by 5 years (Chang TT J Gastroenterol Hepatol 2004: 19:1276–1282)	Good
Adefovir dipivoxil	Interferes with HBV DNA polymerase by chain termination	Yes [48]	No	Yes	Less potent than lamivudine in adult trials More effective than placebo in children aged 12–17 years but not in children aged 2–11 years [48]	Less resistance than lamivudine but 30% by 4 years [102]	Good but need to monitor creatinine as renal tubular acidosis can occur Rate of side-effects similar to placebo in children [48]
Entecavir	Inhibits HBV DNA priming Inhibits reverse transcription of negative-stranded DNA Inhibits synthesis of positive -stranded HBV DNA [51]	In progress	Approved >16 years of age	Yes	More potent than lamivudine and adefovir	Rare [103]	Good

Tenofovir	Selectively inhibits HBV DNA polymerase-reverse-transcriptase in vitro [56]	No (tenofovir has been used in children with HIV)	No	Yes [58]	More potent than adefovir [58]	None reported yet [58]	Similar to adefovir Decreased bone mineral density in children with HIV [56]
Telbivudine	May cause chain termination	No	No	Yes [104]	More potent than lamivudine [104]	Increases with duration of therapy (5% at 1 year and 25% after 2 years [105])	Good Elevation of creatinine can occur [10]

Prolonged treatment with lamivudine increases the risk for emergence of mutation in the HBV polymerase gene at the YMDD locus. This mutation arises because of a methionine-to-valine or a methionine-to-isoleucine switch in the C domain of the HBV polymerase [37]. YMDD variants of HBV are associated with reemergence of active hepatitis or decompensation of chronic liver disease. Once lamivudine therapy is stopped, wild-type virus reappears [38].

There are a number of studies demonstrating lamivudine benefits in children. The first was a double-blind, placebo-controlled, randomized, multi-center study of lamivudine at a dose of 3 mg/kg/day (maximum dose 100 mg) for 52 weeks in 191 children aged 2–17 years compared to placebo in 97 children. All children in the study were HBeAg positive, and had detectable HBV DNA and elevated ALT values. Of those treated with lamivudine, 23% (44/191) cleared HBV DNA and HBeAg compared to 13% (12/97) in the placebo group ($P<0.05$) [39]. Unfortunately, 19% (31/166) developed drug-resistant YMDD mutants. Higher response rates were observed in those with higher ALT levels, as had been noted with IFN. In an open label study of lamivudine in 29 adolescents and young adults with maternally transmitted chronic HBV infection in Taiwan, only those with ALT more than five times the ULN demonstrated a better response (undetectable HBV DNA, normal ALT, and HBeAg/anti-HBe seroconversion) than control patients after 52 weeks of treatment [40].

The optimum duration of lamivudine therapy was investigated in a multi-center, open label study of prolonged therapy in children [41] who had participated in the previous 1 year study of lamivudine [39]. Children were enrolled into one of two groups on the basis of their virological status at week 48 of the original study. A total of 213 children were still HBeAg positive; 133 had received lamivudine and 77 placebo, all were offered lamivudine for a further 2 years. At the end of the study, 51 more children had achieved virological response. However, 100/173 had developed YMDD mutant HBV. The virological response in those with YMDD mutants was only 5% (5/100) compared to 49% (34/70) in those with wild-type HBV. Sixty-three children who were HBeAg negative after the randomized trial (49 previously treated with lamivudine and 14 with placebo) were observed for 2 more years. At the end of the study period, 48/54 (89%) had durable virological responses.

Based on the observation that both therapeutic responses and development of resistant mutants increase in frequency with treatment time, the optimal duration of lamivudine therapy has not been defined. In adults, this agent has largely been replaced by newer drugs with more favorable resistance profiles.

Selecting the children most likely to benefit from lamivudine remains a challenge. Those most likely to have a sustained virological response to lamivudine are those with HBeAg-positive chronic hepatitis and aminotransferases twice the upper limit of normal. If YMDD mutants emerge, lamivudine should be discontinued and liver enzymes need to be monitored. In patients with advanced liver disease, alternate therapy may need to be provided. No serious side effects of lamivudine were reported in children [39]. Lamivudine is excreted by the kidneys; the dose should therefore be reduced in patients with renal failure. Because lamivudine is so well tolerated, many patients, including those with advanced liver disease in whom IFN is contraindicated, can be considered for treatment. Researchers have suggested that the medication should be continued until HBeAg disappears from the serum, anti-HBe appears, or, if neither occurs, HBV DNA becomes persistently undetectable. Most providers continue treatment for at least 6 and up to 12 months after HBeAg seroconversion as "consolidation" of the virological response. It may be prudent to discontinue this agent in children who do not have virological response (disappearance of HBV DNA from serum) after 24 weeks, to minimize the risk of resistance to this and related antiviral agent. In the unusual circumstance of a child with advanced liver disease, addition of another agent may be necessary, if available.

Upon cessation of therapy in adults, 25% of treated patients had elevation of serum ALT of up to three times the baseline, compared with 8% of placebo-treated patients. This "lamivudine withdrawal flare" may progress to jaundice and incipient liver failure, as noted in 2 of 41 patients in a Dutch study [42]. Therefore, monitoring patients for several months after a course of lamivudine is recommended.

Combination therapy with IFN-α and lamivudine has been studied in both children and adults. A pilot study of IFN-α and lamivudine in children with perinatally acquired chronic hepatitis B infection was reported from the UK. This was an open label, single treatment arm, single-center study. IFN-α was used, and the children selected were traditionally regarded as poor responders to treatment. Twenty-three children, all infected in the first year of life, HBeAg positive, and with normal aminotransferases, were treated with lamivudine alone for 8 weeks followed by lamivudine plus IFN-α 5 MU/m^2 three times weekly for 10 months. Of the 23, 5 seroconverted to anti-HBe and 4 of these 5 became HBsAg negative and HBsAb positive. No child developed a YMDD mutant and most (78%) became HBV DNA negative. A side effect of treatment was decrease in weight and linear growth rate, and this remained significant for height 12 months after the end of treatment [43]. In adults with HBeAg-positive chronic HBV, peginterferon α_{2a} alone or peginterferon with lamivudine for 48 weeks was superior to lamivudine alone [44]. Newer nucleoside analogs have displaced lamivudine, so additional combination therapy trials are expected.

Adefovir dipivoxil is a synthetic nucleotide analog of adenosine monophosphate [45]. It suppresses HBV in both HBeAg-positive and negative adults, and drug resistance is lower and emerges later compared to that in lamivudine. In a study of adults with HBeAg-negative chronic HBV, adefovir dipivoxil decreased HBV DNA and aminotransferase levels with prolonged treatment (144 weeks) [46]. When treatment was withdrawn in one subgroup after 48 weeks, the virological and biochemical benefits were lost, suggesting that long-term treatment is required for viral suppression in those with HBeAg-negative chronic hepatitis B infection. Unlike lamivudine, prolonged administration of adefovir led to infrequent development of resistance (5.9% after 144 weeks). Adefovir can be used in patients who have developed YMDD mutants on lamivudine treatment. In a double-blind, randomized trial of 480 HBeAg-positive adults in China, suppression of HBV DNA was observed in those receiving adefovir 10 mg daily for 52 weeks regardless of whether they had wild-type or YMDD mutant infection [45].

Adefovir has been studied in children. Pharmacokinetics as well as safety of adefovir in children and adolescents was reported in a study by Sokal et al. [47]. Adefovir was rapidly absorbed and well tolerated. The dose required to reach exposure similar to that of adults receiving 10 mg/day depended on age: 2–6 years 0.3 mg/kg, 7–11 years 0.25 mg/kg, and 10 mg/day in adolescents. A total of 173 children were recruited for a 48-week multi-center trial of the safety and efficacy of adefovir in children. Of these, 97 had had prior treatment [48]. The children were randomized on a 2:1 basis to adefovir and placebo, and also stratified into three age groups: 2–6 years ($n=35$), 7–11 years ($n=55$), and 12–17 years ($n=83$). Treatment was administered for 48 weeks and the primary endpoints were HBV DNA<1,000 copies/ml and normal ALT at 48 weeks. In adolescents aged 12–17 years, outcomes were similar to those reported in adults. It is unclear why treatment was not as successful in younger children; small numbers and higher baseline HBV DNA levels may have contributed. Adefovir was well tolerated and reported illnesses were judged to be unrelated to the study drug but rather to common childhood conditions. No previously described adefovir treatment associated mutations emerged. Based on this study, adefovir was licensed in USA for children 12–17 years of age. As with other medications in this class, discontinuation may be indicated if there is no virological response after 24 weeks, so that the risk of development of resistance can be limited. As for lamivudine, patients should be monitored for hepatitis flares with drug discontinuation.

Entecavir (ETV) is a cyclopentyl guanosine analog that inhibits HBV polymerase [33]. Entecavir for 48 weeks suppresses HBV DNA viral loads in both HBeAg-positive and negative adults at higher rates compared to lamivudine [49]. Entecavir is also of use in adults with lamivudine refractory HBeAg-positive chronic hepatitis B infection, but a higher dose is required. A 48-week course of entecavir lead to more improvements in histology, viral load reduction, and ALT normalization compared to lamivudine [50]. Entecavir and lamivudine share similar safety profiles except that very high doses of entecavir (30–40 times the usual dose) were associated with brain, pulmonary, and liver tumors in mice. None have been reported in clinical use in humans [51]. Entecavir resistance is rare in treatment-naïve patients [52] even after 5 years [53], and this drug can be used in lamivudine- or adefovir-resistant HBV [51]. Like lamivudine, entecavir appears to be safe in decompensated HBV cirrhosis in adults [54, 55]. Entecavir is available in tablet and suspension forms but is not yet licensed in children less than 16 years of age. A phase II pharmacokinetic and safety trial is in progress, and a phase III trial is planned.

Tenofovir is an oral nucleotide analog, which is similar to adefovir and has significant activity against HBV. It is a potent inhibitor of HBV DNA polymerase-reverse transcriptase in vitro [56]. It also inhibits viral polymerases by direct binding and incorporation into DNA. This is in turn leads to termination of the DNA chain [57]. In adults, tenofovir was found to be more potent (greater decrease in HBV DNA levels) and act more rapidly than adefovir. Interestingly, histological response rates and HBeAg seroconversion rates were similar (21% vs. 18%). Viral suppression rates were high in those who received tenofovir; 80%

of HBeAg-positive patients and 95% of HBeAg-negative patients at week 48 [58]. Although HBsAg seroconversion was uncommon, it was seen more frequently with tenofovir than with adefovir therapy. Resistance did not emerge in a 2-year trial [58]. Tenofovir has demonstrated efficacy in patients with lamivudine and adefovir resistance [59] which persists to up to 5 years of therapy [60]. Tenofovir is currently being tested in a clinical trial in adolescents with chronic HBV.

Chronic Hepatitis B and Organ Transplantation

Children with HBV rarely need a liver transplant for either acute liver failure or decompensated chronic liver disease [61]. Of 215 children who underwent transplantation between 1986 and 1992 at a major French center, only four had HBV-associated disease [62].

HBV infection is the fourth most common cause of acute liver failure in adults in USA [63]. Transplantation is indicated in this setting, since the infection has often been controlled by the time liver failure occurs. Acute liver failure in children is very rarely attributed to HBV.

Chronic HBV infection was a relative contraindication to liver transplantation in the 1970s and 1980s, but the demonstration in the 1990s that administration of Hepatitis B immune globulin (HBIG) is efficacious in decreasing infection of the allograft has allowed successful transplantation with control of re-infection. Success rates were further improved by the addition of lamivudine, so that the outcome of liver transplantation for chronic hepatitis B is now comparable to that for other etiologies in adults [64]. HBIG is expensive and the optimum dose and duration of therapy are unclear. The preferred nucleoside regimen has not been elucidated.

HBV infection can be transmitted via donor livers, and all donors are tested for HBsAg and anti-HBc. Even if anti-HBc is the only positive test, it is recommended that such donor organs should be used only for recipients who already have HBV infection and will receive long-term anti-viral prophylaxis in any case, or for recipients who give informed consent and are also willing to use anti-viral prophylaxis [65].

The course of HBV infection in non-liver solid organ transplant recipients has been examined in a number of ways. In a French study, in which 69 of 874 heart transplant patients were infected with HBV, most through nosocomial infection, chronic HBV infection had little impact on 5-year survival [66]. In a group of 120 lung transplant recipients in Israel, 11 patients with either pre-existing chronic HBV infection or receipt of an organ from an anti-HBc-positive donor were treated with lamivudine prophylaxis. The drug was well tolerated and only one patient developed resistance which responded to a change to adefovir [67]. In Taiwan, overall patient and allograft survival after kidney transplantation was not affected by HBV infection, despite increased hepatic morbidity [68]. Overall, however, the 5-year survival was not dissimilar in those infected with HBV and those uninfected. Lamivudine was used just before and after transplantation in four Chinese adolescents with chronic HBV infection who required renal transplants. Immunosuppression was achieved with prednisolone, cyclosporine A, and mycophenolate mofetil. Three of the four had detectable HBV DNA levels post-transplant but all had normal ALT values and liver function at follow-up, 11–34 months later [69].

Treatment post-solid organ transplant needs to be individualized depending on viral load and the presence or absence of drug resistance conferring viral mutations [70]. Guidelines have been published, but treatment needs of each patient are very different depending on previous therapy, presence or absence of HBV-resistant mutants, and the level of HBV DNA at the time of transplant [71]. Most experts agree that treatment is indicated, at least temporarily, around the time of solid organ or stem cell transplantation, and during immunosuppressive chemotherapy.

Chronic HBV Infections and Renal Disease

Two categories of renal diseases may be associated with chronic HBV in children: children with end stage renal disease who develop nosocomial HBV infection, and patients with chronic HBV who develop membranous glomerulonephropathy leading to nephrotic syndrome. This latter condition leads to end-stage renal disease in 1.4–2.8% of affected children [72], but in adults the course of HBV-associated nephropathy is much less benign. In one series from Hong Kong, 29% of patients developed progressive renal failure and 10% required dialysis during a mean follow-up period of 60 months [73]. The presence of proteinuria mirrors that of HBeAg and usually resolves within 6 months of the loss of HBeAg. Interferon α_{2b} [74, 75] has been used successfully, as has lamivudine [76].

Historically, contaminated hemodialysis equipment, blood transfusions, and blood products were all implicated in the nosocomial transmission of HBV in patients with chronic renal disease. This link was reported in 1975 by a group in USA which reported HBsAg positivity in 36/62 children attending a hemodialysis unit over a 3.5-year period [77]. Screening for prevention of transmission of HBV is now standard for all blood products and donated human tissue. Improved risk management of dialysis equipment and processing has further reduced but not eliminated the risk transmission of HBV in this setting. Immunization against HBV is now recommended in children with renal disease and can be effective [78]. However, patient anti-HBs levels must be tested 1–2 months after the third dose of vaccine. If anti-HBs levels are protective (>10 mIU/mL), then the patient is protected. Titers need to be checked annually and a booster may be required. If anti-HBs is less than 10 mIU/mL after the primary vaccine series, the patient should receive a further three doses and antibody levels should be rechecked [79]. If there is still no response, the child is vulnerable to HBV infection and should be counseled accordingly.

A group of 34 children from Poland with a number of different renal diseases and chronic HBV infection ($N=30$) or chronic HBV and HCV co-infections ($N=4$)

were treated between 1994 and 2002 with different forms of interferon; 14/34 seroconverted to anti-HBe. Duration of follow-up was not reported and there was no control group, but seroconversion rates were encouraging [80]. Oral nucleos(t) ide agents, lamivudine, adefovir, and entecavir, have been used in adults being treated with hemodialysis or after kidney transplantation. Doses need to be adjusted for renal failure and renal function should be monitored closely [70]. The outcome for HBV-infected children with renal disease, treated or untreated, is not yet clear and they will need to be followed for many years. Prevention of HBV infection in this very vulnerable group is key to tackling the impact of HBV on chronic renal disease.

HBV and Hepatitis D Virus Co-infection

Hepatitis D virus (HDV) can only be found in those infected with hepatitis B, as it requires the presence of HBsAg to produce infectious virus particles [81]. Co-infection with HBV and HDV is the commonest in Mediterranean Europe but has been reported from many different global regions. Both acute and chronic HDV infection can lead to the development of rapidly progressive liver disease. Treatment is difficult as there are no specific inhibitors of HDV, and agents that specifically inhibit HBV display little or no activity against HDV. In an Italian multi-center study reported in 1996, treatment with IFN-α_{2b} for either 12 or 24 months in 26 children resulted in only transient improvements in virological and histological endpoints [82]. Similar lack of efficacy was reported in seven children treated in Greece [83]. However, in adults, followed over a 28-year period, HBV replication was associated with increased risk of development of HCC but HDV replication was the only predictor of liver-related mortality [84]. Small studies have demonstrated activity of peginterferon in treatment of chronic HDV [81], but larger studies are required. The optimal duration of IFN therapy is unclear, but if a patient responds, IFN should be maintained at the highest dose tolerated until HDV RNA and HBsAg disappear [81]. There is no evidence yet that combination therapy of lamivudine with IFN or peginterferon offers any advantage over monotherapy with IFN-α alone [85].

Hepatitis C and B Virus Co-infection

Hepatitis B and hepatitis C virus (HCV) infections can occur in the same child as they share the same modes of transmission. Co-infections have been reported in children who received blood transfusions and blood products, such as childhood cancer survivors [86, 87] and children with membranous nephropathy [88]. Adolescents may contract HBV and HCV through intravenous drug use or sexual activity.

In adults, chronic HCV infection even in the setting of co-infection of HBV appears to respond at similar rates to treatment with peginterferon and ribavirin [70]. The situation is not yet clear in children. There are two reports of treatment of children co-infected with HBV and HCV after treatment for childhood malignancies. The most recent paper reported six children aged 8–14 years in Turkey who were treated with IFN-α_{2b} and ribavirin for 12 months. HBV DNA and HCV RNA levels decreased in five and became undetectable in one. This child also seroconverted to anti-HBe and maintained viral suppression [86]. In an older series from Italy, 32 co-infected children previously treated for childhood cancer were followed for a median period of 14 years. Six children spontaneously seroconverted to anti-HBe and also cleared HCV RNA, eight became HBeAg negative but remained HCV RNA positive, and five remained HBeAg positive and became HCV RNA negative. Twelve of thirteen children who were HBeAg and HCV RNA positive were treated with IFN; six had no response, one cleared HBeAg and HCV RNA, one cleared HBeAg but remained HCV RNA positive, and four remained HBeAg positive and cleared HCV RNA. Intriguingly, the response rate of HCV RNA clearance was higher in those co-infected with HBV compared to that in those with HCV infection alone [89].

Chronic HBV and Human Immunodeficiency Virus Co-infection

These infections share common pathways of transmission and are not uncommonly found together in patients. The mortality from HBV is increased in those co-infected with HIV compared to that in those infected with either virus alone [90]. Children co-infected with HIV and HBV have been reported worldwide, some have an underlying condition such as hemophilia [91, 92] while others have unknown modes of acquisition [93]. AIDS-related immunosuppression can reactivate chronic hepatitis B [94] and appears to decrease the rate of spontaneous HBeAg seroconversion. Co-infection makes treatment planning for either infection complex for a number of reasons. Chronic HBV infections can increase the risk of liver toxicity with highly active antiretroviral therapy (HAART) [94]. Co-infected adults may be treated with IFN or non-HIV active anti-HBV nucleoside therapy such as telbivudine or adefovir, or early introduction of HAART. These decisions depend on the status of the HIV infection [95]. The majority of co-infected patients are in resource-poor regions of the world and lamivudine is the only anti-HBV agent readily available. Tenofovir, with its both anti-HIV and HBV properties, may be used in combination with lamivudine to treat chronic HBV alongside HAART therapy [94]. Ideally, oral nucleoside HBV agents are continued indefinitely once HBV DNA is suppressed or for 6 months after anti-HBe develops. Unfortunately, resistance to lamivudine develops in co-infected patients at a rate of 20% of patients per year [96]. When resistance develops, patients are at risk of acute hepatitis flare. Monotherapy of HBV should be avoided as there is a high risk of HIV resistance in addition to HBV resistance [94]. Treatment options in co-infected children are even less clear and must be individualized to take account of the phase of HBV infection (i.e., immune tolerant), HIV activity, drug options, and other confounders such as availability of psycho-social supports.

Summary

The child with chronic hepatitis B most likely to be treated successfully with today's agents is one who displays evidence of immune responsiveness to HBV with elevated ALT levels and at least moderate inflammatory changes on liver biopsy. The child ideally has no other medical problems, and the child and family can comply with the regimen and monitoring.

Even if the child has some success with treatment but remains HBsAg positive, the child is still at risk for HCC or reactivation of hepatitis. If the child is HBsAg negative after treatment, HBV can still be found in the liver and there remains a risk of HCC. Follow-up is required for all children and adults who have ever had chronic hepatitis B infection. We suggest yearly follow-up of virological response, alpha fetoprotein levels, and liver ultrasound for cancer surveillance. This interval should be reduced to 6 monthly if significant fibrosis or cirrhosis is present [97]. The most recent guidelines from AASLD regarding HCC state that all hepatitis B carriers with cirrhosis, regardless of age, should be screened for HCC. Surveillance is also recommended for hepatitis B carriers with a family history of HCC, certain ethnic and age groups, and then individualized depending on current and past hepatic inflammatory disease [98].

Treatment of chronic hepatitis B infection in children, like in adults, is changing to a long-term process, with growth and natural history increasing the complexity of treatment decisions. The availability of new therapeutic agents, higher immunization rates, and heightened surveillance of HCC will hopefully reduce the burden of disease that chronic hepatitis B infection will bring in future years.

References

1. Lok AS, McMahon BJ. Chronic hepatitis B. Hepatology 2007;45:507–539.
2. Degertekin B, Lok ASF. Indications for therapy in hepatitis B. Hepatology 2009; 49:S129–S137.
3. Tillmann HL, Hadem J, Leifeld L, Zachou K, Canbay A, Eisenbach C, Graziadei I, Encke J, Schmidt H, Vogel W, Schneider A, Spengler U, Gerken G, Dalekos GN. Safety and efficacy of lamivudine in patients with severe acute or fulminant hepatitis B, a multicenter experience. J Viral Hepat 2006;13:256–263.
4. Kumar M, Satapathy S, Monga R, Das K, Hissar C, Pande B, Sharma C, Sarin SK. A randomized controllled trial of lamivudine to treat acute hepatitis B. Hepatology 2007;45:97–101.
5. Saldanha J, Gerlich W, Lelie N, Dawson P, Heerman K, Heath A. An international collaborative study to establish a World Health Organization international standard for hepatitis B virus DNA nucleic acid amplification techniques. Vox Sang 2001;80:63–71.
6. Hoofnagle JH. Challenges in therapy of chronic hepatitis B. J Hepatol 2003;39:S230–S235.

7. Iorio R, Pensati P, Botta S, Moschella S, Impagliazzo N, Vajro P, Vegnente A. Side effects of alpha-interferon therapy and impact on health-related quality of life in children with chronic viral hepatitis. Pediatr Infect Dis J 1997;16:984–990.
8. Chang MH, Chen CJ, Lai MS, Hsu HM, Wu TC, Kong MS, Liang DC, Shau WY, Chen DS. Universal hepatitis B vaccination in Taiwan and the incidence of hepatocellular carcinoma in children. Taiwan Childhood Hepatoma Study Group. N Engl J Med 1997;336:1855–1859.
9. Andersson KI, Chung RT. Monitoring during and after antiviral therapy for hepatitis B. Hepatology 2009;49:S166–S173.
10. Huang SN, Chen TC, Tsai SL, Liaw YF. Histopathology and pathobiology of hepatropic virus-induced liver injury. J Gastroenterol Hepatol 1997;12:S195–S217.
11. Knodell RG, Ishak KG, Black WC, Chen TS, Craig R, Kaplowitz N, Kiernan TW, Wollman J. Formulation and application of a numerical scoring system for assessing histological activity in asymptomatic chronic active hepatitis. Hepatology 1981;1:431–435.
12. Batts K, Ludwig J. Chronic hepatitis: an update on terminology and reporting. Am J Surg Pathol 1995;19:1409–1417.
13. Rozario R, Ramakrishna B. Histopathological study of chronic hepatitis B and C: a comparison of two scoring systems. J Hepatol 2003;38:223–229.
14. Sobaniec-Lotowska ME, Lebensztejn D. Histological outcome of chronic hepatitis B in children treated with interferon alpha. World J Gastroenterol 2006;11:7179–7182.
15. Woynarowski M, Cielecka-Kuszyk J, Kaluzynski A, Omulecka A, Sobaniec-Lotowska M, Stolarczyk J, Szczepanski W. Inter-observer variability in histopathological assessment of liver biopsies taken in a pediatric open label therapeutic program for chronic HBV infection treatment. World J Gastroenterol 2006;12:1713–1717.
16. Lebensztejn D, Skiba E, Tobolczyk J, Sobaniec-Lotowska M, Kaczmarski M. Diagnostic accuracy of serum biochemical fibrosis markers in children with chronic hepatitis B evaluated but receiver operating characteristics analysis. World J Gastroenterol 2005;11:7192–7196.
17. Lee WM. hepatitis B virus infection. N Engl J Med 1997;337:1733–1745.
18. Greenberg HB, Pollard RB, Lutwick LI, et al. Effects of human leucocyte interferon and hepatitis B virus infection in patients with chronic active hepatitis. N Engl J Med 1976;295:517–522.
19. Torre D, Tambini R. Interferon-alpha therapy for chronic hepatitis B in children: a meta-analysis. Clin Infect Dis 1996;23:131–137.
20. Sokal EM, Conjeevaram HS, Roberts EA, Alvarez F, Bern E, Goyens P, Rosenthal P, Lachaux A, Shelton M, Sarles J, Hoofnagle J. Interferon alfa therapy for chronic hepatitis B in children: a multinational randomized controlled trial. Gastroenterology 1998;114:988–995.
21. Vajro P, Tedesco M, Fontanella A, DeVincenzo A, Vecchione R, Ammendola R, et al. Prolonged and high dose recombinant interferon alpha-2b alone or after prednisone priming accelerates termination of active viral replication in children with chronic hepatitis B infection. Pediatr Infect Dis J 1996;15:223–231.
22. Lai CL, Lok AS, Lin HJ, et al. Placebo-controlled trial of recombinant alpha2-interferon in Chinese HBsAg-carrier children. Lancet 1987;2:877–880.
23. Lin SM, Sheen IS, Chien RN, Chu CM, Liaw YF. Long-term beneficial effect of interferon therapy in patients with chronic hepatitis B virus infection. Hepatology 1999;29:971–975.
24. Kocak N, Gurakan F, Slatik IN, Ozen H, Yuce A. Long term prognosis of interferon nonresponder children with hepatitis B. Am J Gastroenterol 2000;95:1841.
25. Vo Thi Diem H, Bourgois A, Bontems P, Goyens P, Buts JP, Nackers F, Tonglet R, Sokal EM. Chronic hepatitis B infection: long term comparison of children receiving interferon alpha and untreated controls. J Pediatr Gastroenterol Nutr 2005;40:141–145.
26. Soderstrom A, Lindh M, Ekholm K, Conradi N, Horal P, Krantz M, Hultgren C, Norkrans G. Predictive factors and virological response to interferon treatment in children with chronic hepatitis B. Scand J Infect Dis 2005;37:40–47.
27. Hsu H-Y, Tsai H-Y, Wu T-C, Chiang C-L, Ni y-h, Chen P-J, Chang M-H. Interferon-alpha treatment in children and adults with chronic hepatitis B: a long-term follow-up study in Taiwan. Liver International 2008;28:1288–1297.

28. Vajro P, Migliaro F, Fontanella A, Orso G. Interferon: a meta-analysis of published studies in pediatric chronic hepatitis B. Acta Gastroenterol Belg 1998;61:219–223.
29. van Zonneveld M, Honkoop P, Hansen BE, Niesters HGM, Darwish Murad S, de Man RA, Schalm SW, Janssen HLA. Long term follow-up of alpha-interferon treatment of patients with chronic hepatitis B. Hepatology 2004;39:804–810.
30. Sokal EM. Viral hepatitis throughout infancy to adulthood. Acta Gastroenterol Belg 1998;61:170–174.
31. Giacchino R, Main J, Timitilli A, Giambartolomei G, Facco F, Cirillo C, Jacyna MR, Brook MG, Callea F, Kariayannis P, et al. Dual-centre, double-blind, randomised trial of lymphoblastoid interferon alpha with or without steroid pretreatment in children with chronic hepatitis B. Liver 1995;15:143–148.
32. Kendirli T, Kismet E, Demirkaya E, Aydin HI, Kesik V, Koseoglu V. Death possibly associated with interferon use in a patient with chronic hepatitis. Acta Paediatr 2005;94:984–985.
33. Loomba R, Liang TJ. Novel approaches to new therapies for hepatitis B virus infection. Antivir Ther 2006;11:1–15.
34. Fontana R. side effects of long-term oral antiviral therapy for hepatitis B. Hepatology 2009;49:S185–S195.
35. Lai C-L, Chien R-N, Leung NWY, Chang T-T, Guan R, Tai D-I, et al. A one-year trial of lamivudine for chronic hepatitis B. N Engl J Med 1998;339:61–68.
36. Dienstag JL, Schiff ER, Wright TL, Perillo RP, Hann H-WL, Goodman Z, et al. Lamivudine as initial treatment for chronic hepatitis B in the United States. N Engl J Med 1999;341:1256–1263.
37. Tipples GA, Ma MM, Fischer KP, Bain VG, Kneteman NM, Tyrrell DLJ. Mutation in HBV RNA-dependent DNA polymerase confers resistance to lamivudine *in vivo*. Hepatology 1996;24:714–717.
38. Fontana R. Antivirals in hepatitis B. Clin Perspect Gastroenterol 1999:207–213.
39. Jonas MM, Kelley DA, Mizerski J, Badia IB, Areias JA, Schwarz KB, Little NR, Greensmith MJ, Gardner SD, Bell MS, Sokal EM. Clinical trial of lamivudine in children with chronic hepatitis B. N Engl J Med 2002;346:1706–1713.
40. Alexander G, Baba CS, Chetri K, Negi TS, Choudhuri G. High rates of early HBeAg seroconversion and relapse in Indian patients of chronic hepatitis B treated with lamivudine: results of an open labeled trial. BMC Gastroenterol 2005;5:29.
41. Sokal EM, Kelly DA, Mizerski J, Badia IB, Areias JA, Schwarz KB, Vegnente A, Little NR, Gardener SD, Jonas MM. Long-term lamivudine therapy for children with HBeAg-positive chronic hepatitis B. Hepatology 2006;43:225–232.
42. Honkoop P, De Man RA, Niesters HG, Zondervan PE, Schalm SW. Acute exacerbation of chronic hepatitis B virus infection after withdrawal of lamivudine therapy. Hepatology 2000;32:635–639.
43. D'Antiga L, Aw M, Atkins M, Moorat A, Vergani D, Mieli-Vergani G. Combined lamivudine/interferon-alpha treatment in "immunotolerant" children perinatally infected with hepatitis B: a pilot study. J Pediatr 2006;148:228–233.
44. Lau GK, Piratvisuth T, Luo KX, Marcellin P, Thongsawat S, Cooksley G, Gane E, Fried MW, Chow WC, Paik SW, Chang WY, Berg T, Flisiak R, McCloud P, Pluck N. Peginterferon Alfa-2a, lamivudine, and the combination for HBeAg-positive chronic hepatitis B. N Engl J Med 2005;352:2682–2695.
45. Zeng M, Mao Y, Yao G, Wang H, Hou J, Wang Y, Ji BN, Chang CN, Barker KF. A double-blind randomized trial of adefovir dipivoxil in Chinese subjects with HBeAg-positive chronic hepatitis B. Hepatology 2006;44:108–116.
46. Hadziyannis SJ, Tassopoulos NC, Heathcote EJ, Chang TT, Kitis G, Rizzetto M, Marcellin P, Lim SG, Goodman Z, Ma J, Arterburn S, Xiong S, Currie G, Brosgart CL. Long-term therapy with adefovir dipivoxil for HBeAg-negative chronic hepatitis B. N Engl J Med 2005;352:2673–2681.
47. Jonas MM, Kelly DA, Pollack H, Mizerski J, Sorbel J, Frederick D, Mondou E, Rousseau F, Sokal EM. Safety, efficacy, and pharmacokinetics of adefovir dipivoxil in children and adolescents (age 2 to < 18 years) with chronic hepatitis B. Hepatology 2008;47:1863–1871.

48. Sokal EM, Kelly DA, Wirth S, Dhawan A, Frederick D. The pharmacokinetics and safety of adefovir dipivoxil in children and adolescents with chronic hepatitis B virus infection. J Clin Pharmacol 2008;48:512–517.
49. Lok AS. The maze of treatments for hepatitis B. N Engl J Med 2005;352:2743–2746.
50. Sherman M, Yurdaydin C, Sollano J, Silva M, Liaw YF, Cianciara J, Boron-Kaczmarska A, Martin P, Goodman Z, Colonno R, Cross A, Denisky G, Kreter B, Hindes R. Entecavir for treatment of lamivudine-refractory, HBeAg-positive chronic hepatitis B. Gastroenterology 2006;130:2039–2049.
51. Dienstag J. Benefits and risks of nucleoside analog therapy for hepatitis B. Hepatology 2009;49:S112–S121.
52. Colonno R, Rose RE, Pokornowski K, Baldick CJ, Eggers B, Yu D, Cross A, Tenney DJ. Four year assessment of ETV resistance in nucleoside-naive and lamivudine refractory patients. J Hepatology 2007;46:S294.
53. Chang TT, Lai CL, Yoon SK, Lee SS, Coelho HSM, Carrilho FJ, Poordad F, Halota W, Horsmans Y, Tsai N, Zhang H, Tenney DJ, Tamez R, Iloeje U. Entecavir treatment for up to 5 years in patients hepatitis B e antigen-positive chronic hepatitis B. Hepatology 2010; 51:1–9.
54. Shim JH, Lee HC, Kim KM, Lim Y-S, Chung Y-H, Lee YS, Suh DJ. Efficacy of entecavir in treatment naive patients with hepatitis B virus related decompensated cirrhosis. J Hepatol 2010;52:176–182.
55. Fontana R. Entecavir in decompensated HBV cirrhosis: the future is looking brighter. J Hepatol 2010;52:147–149.
56. Heijtink RA, Kruining J, De Wilde GA, Balzarini J, De Clercq E, Schalm SW. Inhibitory effects of acyclic nucleoside phosphonates on human hepatitis B virus and duck hepatitis B virus infections in tissue culture. Antimicrob Agents Chemother 1994;38:2180–2182.
57. Delaney WE, Ray AS, Yang H, Qi X, Xiong S, Zhu Y, Miller MD. Intracellular metabolism and in vitro activity of tenofovir against hepatitis B virus. Antimicrob Agents Chemother 2006;50:2471–2477.
58. Marcellin P, Heathcote EJ, Buti M, Gane E, De Man RA, Krastev Z, Germanidis G, Lee SS, Flisiak R, Kaita k, Manns M, Kotzev I, Tchernev K, Buggisch P, Weilert F, Ovung Kurdas O, Shiffman ML, Trinh H, Washington MK, Sorbel J, Anderson J, Snow-Lampart A, Mondou E, Quinn J, Rousseau F. Tenofovir disoproxil fumarate versus adefovir dipivoxil for chronic hepatitis B. N Engl J Med 2008;359:2442–2455.
59. van Bommel F, Zollner B, Sarrazin C, Spengler U, Huppe D, Moller B, Feucht H-H, Wiedenmann B, Berg T. Tenofovir for patients with lamivudine-resistant hepatitis B virus (HBV) infection and high HBV DNA level during adefovir therapy. Hepatology 2006;44:318–325.
60. Van Bommel F, De Man RA, Wedemeter H, Deterding K, Petersen J, Buggisch P, Erhardt A, Huppe D, Stein K, Trojan J, Sarrazin C, Bocher W, Spengler U, Wasmuth HE, Reinders JGP, Moller B, Rhode P, Feucht HH, Wiedenmann B, Berg T. Long term efficacy of tenofovir monotherapy for hepatitis B virus-mono-infected patients after failure of nucleoside/nucleotide analogues. Hepatology 2010;51:73–80.
61. Squires R, Shneider B, Bucuvalas J, Alonso E, Sokol R, Narkewicz MR, Dhawan A, Rosenthal P, Baez-Rodriguez N, Murray K, Horslen S, Martin M, Lopez M, Soriano H, McGuire B, Jonas MM, Yazigi N, Shepherd R, Scharz K, Lobritto S, Thomas D, Lavine J, Karpen S, Ng V, Kelly DA, Simonds N, Hynan L. Acute liver failure in children: the first 349 patients in the pediatrics acute liver failure study group. J Pediatr 2006;148: 652–658.
62. Lykavieris P, Fabre M, Yvart J, Alvarez F. HBV infection in pediatric liver transplantation. J Pediatr Gastroenterol Nutr 1993;16:321–327.
63. Ostapowicz G, Fontana R, Scholdt F, Larson A, Davem T, Han S, McCashland T, Sahakil A, Hay E, Hynan L, Crippin J, Blei A, Samuel G, Reisch J, Lee W. Results of a prospective study of acute liver failure at 17 tertiary care centers in the United States. Ann Intern Med 2002;137:947–954.

64. Kim WR, Poteruscha JJ, Kremers WK, Ishitani MB, Dickson ER. Outcome for liver transplantation for hepatitis B in the United States. Liver Transpl Surg 2004;10:968–974.
65. Hoofnagle JH. Reactivation of hepatitis B. Hepatology 2009;49:S156–S165.
66. Lunel F, Cadranel JF, Rosenheim M, Dorent R, Di-Martino V, Payan C, Fretz C, Ghoussoub JJ, Bernard B, Dumont B, Perrin M, Gandjbachkh I, Huraux JM, Stuyver L, Opolon P. Hepatitis virus infections in heart transplant recipients: epidemiology, natural history, characteristics, and impact on survival. Gastroenterology 2000;119:1064–1074.
67. Shitrit A, Kramer M, Bakal I, Morali G, Ari Z, Ari Z, Shitrit D. Lamivudine prophylaxis for hepatits B virus infection after lung transplantation. Ann Thorac Surg 2006;81: 1851–1852.
68. Huo TI, Yang WC, Wu JC, King KL, Loong CC, Lin CY, Lui WY, Chang FY, Lee SD. Impact of hepatitis B and C virus infection on the outcome of kidney transplantation in Chinese patients. Chung Hua I Hsueh Tsa Chih (Taipei) 2000;63:93–100.
69. Lau S, Tse K, Lai W, Chiu M. Use of prophylactic lamivudine and mycophenolare mofetil in renal transplant recipients with chronic hepatitis B infection. Pediatr Transplant 2003;7:376–380.
70. Peters MG. Special populations with hepatitis B virus infection. Hepatology 2009; 49:S146–S155.
71. Coffin CS, Terrault NA. Management of hepatitis B in liver transplant patients. J Viral Hepat 2007;14:37–44.
72. Gilbert RD, Wiggelinkhuizen J. The clinical course of hepatitis B associated nephropathy. Pediatr Nephrol 1994;8:11–14.
73. Lai KN, Li PK, Lui SF, Au TC, Tam JS, Tong KL, Lai FM. Membranous nephropathy related to hepatitis B virus in adults. N Engl J Med 1991;324:1457–1463.
74. Lin CY. Treatment of hepatitis B virus-associated membranous nephropathy with recombinant alpha-interferon. Kidney Int 1995;47:225–230.
75. Jonas MM, Ragin L, Silva MO. Membranous glomerulonephritis and chronic persistent hepatitis B in a child: treatment with recombinant interferon alfa. J Pediatr 1991;119:818–820.
76. Connor FL, Rosenberg AR, Kennedy SE, Bohane TD. HBV associated nephrotic syndrome: resolution with oral lamivudine. Arch Dis Child 2003;88:446–449.
77. Fine RN, Malekzadeh MH, Wright Jr HT. Hepatitis C in a pediatric hemodialysis unit. J Pediatr 1975;86:349–355.
78. Watkins SL, Alexander SR, Brewer ED, Hesley TM, West DJ, Chan ISF, Mendelman P, Bailey SM, Burns JL, Hogg RJ. Response of recombinant hepatitis B vaccine in children and adolescents with chronic renal failure. Am J Kidney Dis 2002;40:365–372.
79. (ACIP) ACoIP. Guidelines for vaccinating kidney dialysis patients and patients with chronic kidney disease. Center for disease control 2006.
80. Szczepanska M, Tobis A, Schneiberg B, Szprynger K, Kobos E, Morawiec-Knysak A. Treatment of chronic hepatitis with interferon in children with kidney diseases. Pol Merkur Lekarski 2005;18:22–28.
81. Farci P, Chessa C, Balestrieri C, Serra G, Lai ME. Treatment of chronic hepatitis D. J Viral Hepat 2007;14 (Suppl 1):58–63.
82. Di Marco V, Giacchino R, Timitilli A, Bortoletti F, Crivellaro C, Calzia R, Iannuzzi C, Prestoleo T, Vajro P, Nebbia G, Stringhi C, Rosina F, Biassoni D, Callaca F. Long-term interferon-α treatment of children with chronic hepatitis delta: a multicentre study. J Viral Hepat 1996;3:123–128.
83. Dalekos GN, Galanakis E, Zervou E, Tzoufi M, Latsanis PD, Tsianos EV. Interferon-alpha treatment of children with chronic hepatitis D virus infection; the Greek experience. Hepatogastroenterology 2000;47:1072–1076.
84. Romeo R, Del Ninno E, Rumi M, Russo A, Sangiovanni A, de Franchis R, Ronchi G, Colombo M. A 28-year study of the course of hepatitis D infection: a risk factor for cirrhosis and hepatocellular carcinoma. Gastroenterology 2009;136:1629–1638.
85. Niro GA, Rosina F, Rizzetto M. Treatment of hepatitis D. J Viral Hepat 2005;12:2–9.

86. Urganci N, Gulec S, Dogan S, Nuhoglu A. Interferon and ribavirin treatment results of patients with HBV-HCV co-infection cured of childhood malignancies. Int J Infect Dis 2006;10:453–457.
87. Utilli R, Zampino, R, Bellopede P, Marracino M, Ragone E, Adinolfi LE, Ruggiero G, Capasso M, Indolfi P, Casale F, Martini A, Di Tullio MT. Dual or single hepatitis B and C virus infections in childhood cancer survivors: long-term follow-up and effect of Interferon treatment. Blood 1999;94:4046–4052.
88. Sithebe NP, Kramvis A, Kew MC, Bhimma R, Coovadia HM, Naidoo P. Hepatitis B and C virus co-infection in black children with membranous nephropathy. Pediatr Nephrol 2002;17:689–694.
89. Utili R, Zampino R, Bellopede P, Marracino M, Ragone E, Adinolfi LE, Ruggiero G, Capasso M, Indolfi P, Casale F, Martini A, Di Tullio MT. Dual or single hepatitis B and C virus infections in childhood cancer survivors: long-term follow-up and effect of interferon treatment. Blood 1999;94:4046–4052.
90. Thio CL, Seaberg EC, Skolasky R, Phair J, Visscher B, Munoz A, Thomas DL. HIV-1, hepatitis B virus, and risk of liver-related mortality in the multicenter cohort study (MACS). Lancet 2002;360:1921–1926.
91. Wagner N, Rotthauwe HW, Becker M, Dienes HP, Mertens T, Fodisch HJ, Brackmann HH. Correlation of hepatitis B virus, hepatitis D virus and human immunodeficiency virus type 1 infection markers in hepatitis B suface antigen positive haemophiliacs and patients without haemophilia with clinical and histopathological outcome of hepatitis. Eur J Pediatr 1992;151:90–94.
92. Kebudi R, Aoluo L, Badur S. The seroprevalence of HIV-1 and HBV infections in multi-transfused pediatric hematology-oncology patients in Istanbul. Pediatr Hematol Oncol 1992;9:389–391.
93. Rouet F, Chaix ML, Inwoley A, Anaky MF, Fassinou P, Kpozehouen C, Blanche S, Msellati P. Frequent occurrence of chronic hepatitis B virus infections among West African HIV type-1 infected children. Clin Infect Dis 2008;46:361–366.
94. Hoffmann CJ, Thio CL. Clinical implications of HIV and hepatitis B co-infections in Asia and Africa. Lancet Infect Dis 2007;7:402–409.
95. Rockstroh JK, Bhagani S, Benhamou Y, Bruno R, Mauss S, Peters L, Puoti M, Soriano V, Tural C. European AIDS clinical society (EACS) guidelines for the clinical management and treatment of chronic hepatitis B and C co-infection in HIV-infected adults. HIV Med (2008);9:82–88.
96. Benhamou Y, Bochet M, Thibault V, Di Martino V, Caumes E, Bricaire F, Opolon P, Katlama C, Poynard T. Long-term incidence of hepatitis B virus resistance to lamivudine in human immunodeficiency virus-infected patients. Hepatology 1999;30:1302–1306.
97. Shah U, Kelly DA, Chang M-H, Fujisawa T, Heller S, Gonzalez-Peralta RP, Jara P, Mieli-Vergani G, Mohan N, Murray K. Management of chronic hepatitis B in Children. J Pediatr Gastroenterol Nutr 2009;48:399–404.
98. Bruix J, Sherman M. Management of hepatocellular carcinoma. Hepatology 2005; 42:1208–1236.
99. Gurakan F, Kocak N, Ozen H, Yuce A. Comparison of standard and high dosage recombinant interferon alpha 2b for treatment of children with chronic hepatitis B infection. Pediatr Infect Dis J 2000;19:52–56.
100. Barbera C, Bortoletti F, Crivellaro C, et al. Recombinant interferon-alpha 2a hastens the rate of HBeAg clearance in children with chronic hepatitis B. Hepatology 1994;20:287–290.
101. Giacchino R, Main J, Timitilli A, Giambartolomei G, Facco F, Cirillo C, et al. Dual-centre, double-blind, randomised trial of lymphoblastoid interferon alpha with or without steroid pretreatment in children with chronic hepatitis B. Liver 1995;15:143–148.
102. Fung SK, Chae HB, Fontana R, Conjeevaram HS, Marrero J, Oberhelman K, Hussain M, Lok AS. Virologic response and resistance to adefovir in patients with chronic hepatitis B. J Hepatol 2006;44:283–290.

103. Colonno RJ, Rose RE, Baldick CJ, Levine S, Pokornowski K, Yu CF, Walsh A, Fang J, Hsu M, Mazzucco C, Eggers B, Zhang S, Plym M, Klesczewski K, Tenney DJ. Entecavir resistance is rare in nucleoside naive patients with hepatitis B. Hepatology 2006;44:1656–1665.
104. Lai CL, Gane E, Liaw Y-F, Hsu C-W, Thongsawat S, Wang YJ, Chen Y-B, Heathcote EJ, Rasenack J, Bzowej N, Naoumov NV, Di Bisceglie AM, Zeuzem S, Moon YM, Goodman Z, Chao G, Fielman Constance B, Brown NA. Telbivudine versus lamivudine in patients with chronic hepatitis B. N Engl J Med (2007);357:2576–2587.
105. Liaw YF, Gane E, Zeuzem S, Wang Y, Heathcote EJ, Manns M, Bzowej N, Niu J, Han SH, Hwang SG, Cakaloglu Y, Tong MJ, Papatheodoridis G, Chen Y, Brown NA, Albanis E, Galil K, Naoumov NV. 2-Year GLOBE trial results: telbivudine is superior to lamivudine in patients with chronic hepatitis B. Gastroenterology 2009;136:486–495.

Epidemiology and Natural History of Hepatitis C in Children

Nanda Kerkar

Key Concepts

- HCV is an RNA virus and while 4.1 million people in the USA are currently positive for antibody to HCV, the incidence of new infections is declining.
- Perinatal transmission is the most common mode of acquiring HCV infection in children.
- Screening of infants for antibody to HCV should be postponed until 18 months of age as maternal antibodies may persist until then.
- Evaluation of children with history of multiple transfusions in the decades before routine screening for HCV has provided useful natural history information.
- The majority of children infected with HCV will go on to develop chronic infection and liver disease of variable severity.

Keywords Incidence • RNA virus • Quasispecies • Genotype • Financial burden • HCV screening • Natural history • Acute HCV • Perinatally acquired HCV • Anti-HCV testing • Immune response • Autoimmunity • High-risk populations • Coinfection with HIV

Introduction

Hepatitis C virus (HCV) is the most common cause of chronic liver disease, cirrhosis, and hepatocellular carcinoma in adults in many parts of the world including the USA. HCV has been recognized as the most common agent associated with posttransfusion non-A, non-B hepatitis. Numerous epidemiologic studies indicate

N. Kerkar (✉)
Mount Sinai School of Medicine, Box 1104, One Gustave L Levy Place, New York, NY, 10029, USA
e-mail: nanda.kerkar@mountsinai.org

M.M. Jonas (ed.), *Viral Hepatitis in Children: Unique Features and Opportunities*, Clinical Gastroenterology, DOI 10.1007/978-1-60761-373-2_4,

that the most efficacious route for HCV transmission is parenteral, blood and blood products, intravenous drug abuse, hemodialysis, organ transplantation and needle-stick injuries. HCV may also be implicated in a proportion of sporadic non-A, non-B hepatitis cases, but sexual transmission is relatively uncommon. In children, perinatal transmission is the most common mode of acquiring HCV infection. Although the incidence of HCV infection remains high, the data from the Center for Disease Control and Prevention show that the incidence of new infections peaked in 1989 at 291,000 and has since been steadily declining, being 17,000 in 2007 (Fig. 1). This dramatic decline correlates with a decrease in acute cases associated with injection drug use, although the reasons are unclear [1]. The fact that clinical disease is apparent in only about 30% of all newly acquired HCV infections may be contributory, making the true incidence higher [2, 3].

Molecular Biology

HCV is a 9.4-kb single-stranded RNA virus belonging to the Flaviviridae family. HCV virus has never been visualized or grown in tissue culture. Given the extremely low titer of HCV in serum, a novel molecular approach was used to identify the virus. Antibodies present in sera of suspected cases were used to screen differen-

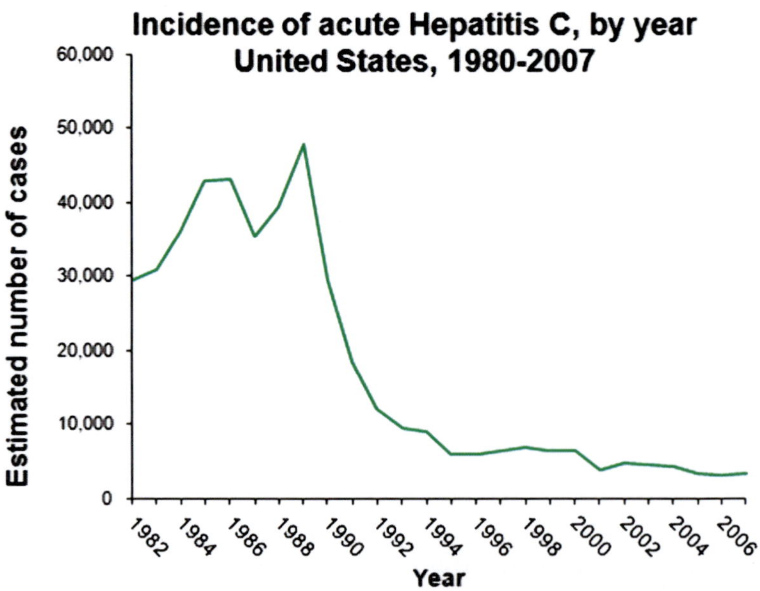

Fig. 1 The incidence of HCV infection in the USA is declining over the years. *Figure obtained from the Centers of Disease Control and Prevention website*

tially an expression cDNA library prepared from relatively high-titer infectious chimpanzee serum [4]. In 1989, the cDNA of the HCV genome was successfully cloned [5]. RNA-dependent polymerases, such as that of HCV, lack the ability to "proofread" during transcription and thus are prone to incorporating erratic nucleotides during viral replication. As a result, HCV is a highly heterogeneous pathogen existing as very closely related genomes called quasispecies [6]. Increased HCV quasispecies heterogeneity correlates with less favorable response to antiviral treatment and possibly with the natural history of infection in children [7, 8]. Assays to assess HCV quasispecies are expensive, not standardized, and not routinely used in clinical practice [9]. Six genotypes [1–6] and about 100 subtypes [10] have been described. Genotypes 1 and 2 have a worldwide distribution, genotype 3 is most common in Australia and the Indian sub-continent, genotypes 4 and 5 are observed in the Middle East and sub-Saharan Africa, and genotype 6 is found mainly in Asia. Genotype 1 accounts for around 75% of all HCV in the USA, genotype 2 for 15%, genotype 3 for 7%, genotype 4 for 1%, and genotype 6 for 3%. Genotypes 1 and 4 are relatively resistant to treatment [1].

Epidemiology

HCV infection affects people of all ages, but most acute cases of hepatitis C occur in young adults. Worldwide, 180 million people are infected with HCV [11]. In the USA approximately 4.1 million persons are positive for antibody to HCV, 80% of whom are reported to be viremic [12]. The prevalence is higher among African Americans (3.2%) and Hispanics (2.1%) than that among non-Hispanic whites [13]. Although death from fulminant HCV is rare, an estimated 8,000–10,000 deaths occur annually from HCV-related chronic liver disease [1] and it is currently the most frequent indication for liver transplantation in the adult population. In the late 1990s, it was projected that there will be a 61% increase in cirrhosis, a 279% increase in decompensated liver disease, 68% increase in hepatocellular carcinoma, and >500% increase for liver transplantation in the following decade [13]. In 1995, there were an estimated 26,700 hospitalizations at a cost of $514 million for inpatient care alone and 2,600 deaths caused by HCV infection in acute nonfederal hospitals in the USA; this extrapolated to a total cost of $1.5 billion in 1995 alone, secondary to HCV-related morbidity [14].

It is believed that HCV reached the USA around 1910 at the conclusion of the Spanish–American war, based on phylogenetic analysis [15, 16]. However, identification of the virus in human subjects was only possible after a specific diagnostic tool for circulating HCV antibody (anti-HCV) was developed using purified viral polypeptide derived from recombinant yeast expressing a small part of the viral genome [5]. The development of an assay to detect HCV led to the initiation of routine screening of blood and organ donors for HCV, and this practice has led to the decline in the prevalence of hepatitis following transfusion and transplantation. The risk factors for HCV infection were quantified in the 1990s as follows: transfusion of blood or blood products 34.4%, intravenous drug abuse 20.6%, heterosexual contact 3.8%, occupational risk 1.9%, and tattoos 0.6% [17]. In the UK, a regional study of blood donors carried out from October 1991 to February 1994 in Ireland identified 14 men and 15 women with HCV antibodies [18]. These 15 women were substantially different from the overall donor pool and 13 (87%) of them were Rh-negative, 12 of whom had received anti-D immune globulin in 1977. In 1994, batches of anti-D immune globulin used in Ireland during 1977 and 1978 to prevent Rh isoimmunization were found to be contaminated with HCV from a single infected donor (genotype 1b). This discovery provoked a major health crisis and a national screening program was established in addition to other measures. Of 62,667 women screened, 390 women were found to be infected with HCV, based on positive HCV RNA, and 376 were available for further screening. Following the course of these women who had been infected with HCV for 17 years allowed some light to be shed on the natural history of HCV, given that they were all infected from a common source. A total of 304 women (81%) reported symptoms, most commonly fatigue, and serum transaminases were slightly elevated (40–899 U/L) in 176 of 371 (47%) and above 100 U/L in 8%. Liver biopsies showed inflammation in 356 of 363 women (98%), inflammation was mild in 47% and moderate in 52%. Although 51% showed evidence of fibrosis, only 2% had probable or definite cirrhosis [18].

Acute HCV

After initial exposure, HCV RNA can be detected in blood in 1–3 weeks. Within an average of 50 days (range 15–150 days), virtually all patients develop liver cell injury as shown by elevation of aminotransferases [19]. Antibody to HCV can be detected in 50–70% of patients at the onset of symptoms and in approximately 90% of patients 3 months after the onset of infection. Clinically, HCV infection in adults appears to have a dichotomous course, where the majority live a normal life span, but a proportion have a severe course. About 15% of HCV-infected adults recover spontaneously, 25% have an asymptomatic illness with persistently abnormal liver enzymes and generally benign histological lesions, and in the remaining 60%, there is biochemical evidence of chronic hepatitis. The majority with chronic hepatitis have mild to moderate necroinflammatory lesions with minimal fibrosis, while 20% develop cirrhosis in 10–20 years and may die of complications if liver transplantation is not available. Fulminant liver failure after HCV has been reported but is extremely rare. Children who are acutely infected with HCV, like adults are generally asymptomatic, but they are more likely than infected adults to spontaneously clear the virus [20]. Approximately 90% of infected children will have abnormal ALT in the first year of life and half of them will have ALT more than two times the upper limit of normal.

Perinatally Acquired HCV

After universal testing of blood donors for anti-HCV was commenced in 1992, mother to child (vertical or perinatal) transmission has replaced transfusion-associated hepatitis C to become the most common mode of HCV transmission among children in the USA [21]. Vertical transmission of HCV may occur in utero, transplacentally at any time during pregnancy, or at the time of delivery. Between 20,000 and 40,000 children in the USA have chronic HCV infection, with 7,200 new cases annually mainly from vertical transmission [22, 23]. The seroprevalence increases with age: 0.2% of children aged 6–11 years and 0.4% of children aged 12–19 years have positive HCV antibodies [23]. The prevalence of HCV infection among women of child-bearing age is 1.2% and is higher in women who are injection drug users or who are HIV coinfected [23, 24]. The risk of perinatal HCV transmission is 4–6% and is two- to threefold higher for mothers with HIV/HCV coinfection. Delivery by cesarean section is not advocated by most obstetricians, although some pediatricians advise against use of fetal scalp monitors and recommend delivery within 6 h of rupture of membranes to avoid transmission when the mother is known to be HCV infected [11]. Although HCV has been identified in breast milk of infected mothers, breastfeeding is not prohibited in HCV-infected mothers. In the USA, horizontal transmission from child to child is rare.

Given that maternal antibodies can migrate across the placenta, establishing a diagnosis of HCV in those with vertically transmitted infection can be problematic. According to current guidelines, anti-HCV testing should be postponed till 18 months of age [23]. If earlier diagnosis is desired, HCV RNA may be performed at or after the child's first well-child visit at 1–2 months of age. However, given that the sensitivity of the test is low at this age, it is prudent to defer the HCV RNA testing till the child is at least 6 months old when the sensitivity of the test is improved [11]. For perinatally acquired HCV, 25% had spontaneous clearance by 7.3 years. Younger age at follow-up and a normal ALT both favored spontaneous viral clearance ($p<0.0001$) [25]. In children with vertically acquired HCV, short-term studies have shown that clinical symptoms are seen in only about 20%, with hepatomegaly being the most common clinical abnormality [26]. Of 70 children, born to HCV-infected women enrolled between 1990 and 1999, 93% had elevated ALT in the first year of life, 19% had sustained ALT normalization with loss of HCV RNA within 30 months of life, and 50% were genotype 3. The cumulative probability of chronic progression was 81%, the chronic infection was asymptomatic and liver disease mild in the 11 children who had liver biopsy [27]. Another multi-center study followed 200 white children with HCV for up to 17.5 years and reported that only 6% achieved sustained viral clearance and normalization of ALT [28]. In 92 liver biopsy specimens, the mean fibrosis score was 1.5 ± SD1.3 for children <15 years of age and 2.3 ± SD1.2 for children >15 years of age. The majority of studies have demonstrated minimal fibrosis and rare cirrhosis 15–20 years after HCV infection [28–30]. A study in 60 children with HCV, in a quarternary referral center serving a multiethnic population in the USA, showed that 12% of children had bridging fibrosis on liver biopsy after a mean duration of infection of 13 years [31]. On follow-up, two patients underwent liver transplantation, one of whom had undiagnosed HCC.

Immune Response and HCV

Approximately 85% of HCV-infected individuals fail to clear the virus by 6 months and develop chronic hepatitis with persistent sometimes intermittent viremia. This ability to produce chronic hepatitis is one of the most striking features of HCV infection and is responsible for the morbidity and mortality associated with this virus. Similar to other viruses, eradication of HCV infection requires efficient innate and adaptive immune responses. A strong multi-specific lymphocyte response, including CD4+ and CD8+ T lymphocytes, NK cells, and B lymphocytes, in association with dendritic cell activity is associated with pathogen clearance and disease resolution [32]. In contrast, a narrowly focused and/or delayed response of T lymphocytes and limited B lymphocyte activation are associated with chronic HCV infection. The mechanism of impaired adaptive immune activation in those who develop chronic HCV infection is not well understood, but an inefficient and fading CD4+ and CD8+ lymphocyte activation seems to be a prevalent factor [33]. Another factor appears to be virus related. Given the intrinsic error rate of viral RNA polymerase, HCV exists in a heterogeneous quasispecies and has a high rate of mutation, hence a lot of attention has been focused on the possibility of immune escape mutation [34]. Cytotoxic T lymphocyte escape mutation was first observed within several months of experimental inoculation in a chimpanzee that subsequently developed chronic HCV infection [35]. It has been reported that the cytotoxic T cell response to an epitope in the hypervariable region of the hepatitis C virus was quantitatively greater (up to tenfold) in patients with HCV clearance than that in those with chronic infection [36]. Currently, it is known that T cells with regulatory capacity are enriched during HCV infection; however, the mechanism by which these regulatory cells influence the immune response in HCV remains to be elucidated. Reinfection with HCV has been demonstrated in animal studies and in humans [37]. Similar to what has been observed in chimpanzees, levels of HCV viremia following reinfection are lower, generally transient, and shorter in duration compared to that in the initial infection [38].

HCV and Autoimmunity

A link between viruses and autoimmunity has been proposed since the immune system was first found to be capable of attacking self-components, the classical view being that a viral infection precedes and triggers autoimmune responses. The first suggestion that HCV may be linked to autoimmunity stems from the observation that liver kidney microsomal (LKM) antibody, which is seen in type 2 autoimmune hepatitis, is at times present in patients with chronic HCV [39]. Persuasive evidence that infection with HCV can lead directly to autoimmunity is provided in three key papers. In the first, it was demonstrated that short amino acid sequences are shared in common between cytochrome P4502D6, the target of LKM in autoimmune hepatitis, and the HCV polyprotein [40]. This suggests that molecular mimicry may be the mechanism triggering liver-specific autoimmunity. In the second paper, temporal relationship was demonstrated between HCV infection and development of LKM, giving support to the concept that the two may be causally related. A child started producing LKM 2 weeks after being infected by HCV following liver transplantation for end-stage liver disease secondary to alpha-1 antitrypsin deficiency [41]. The production of LKM was initially of IgM subtype, then both IgM and IgG, and thereafter solely IgG. In the third paper, there is report of LKM-positive autoimmune hepatitis developing in a nurse with a predisposing HLA haplotype who had a needlestick injury while caring for a HCV-infected patient [42]. Experiments using LKM-positive sera showing cross-reactivity with both cytochrome P450D6, the target of LKM, and an epitope on HCV have also been reported; the two epitopes shared sequence homology [43]. The clinical relevance of finding positive autoimmune markers in HCV is that necroinflammatory flares may be observed in a proportion of patients treated with anti-viral therapy who will require careful monitoring and treatment with corticosteroids [44].

Natural History

There are few published data regarding the epidemiology and natural history of HCV infection, especially in children. Acute hepatitis and biochemical evidence of hepatic injury are common in recipients of multiple transfusions for thalassemia, leukemia, and hemophillia. A study in 1991 reported detection of anti-HCV antibodies in 95% of hemophiliac children aged 1–10 years who had received untreated factor concentrates [45]. The rate of HCV positivity was higher than that in several studies of adult hemophiliacs (59–80%), and may relate to the severity of the disease and the need for multiple factor transfusions [46]. Other researchers also detected HCV viremia by PCR and found that it correlated with abnormal transaminase levels [47]. Although there was no histological assessment of liver injury in either study, reports from adult studies indicate that cirrhosis may occur in 15% of adult hemophiliacs [48]. A pediatric study following 78 children who had received multiple transfusions secondary to thalassemia for 13 years reported that 80% of the children were diagnosed with acute or chronic non-A, non-B hepatitis [49] and 56% of those positive for HCV developed a chronic course. Another study reported an occurrence of acute non-A, non-B hepatitis in 61% of children with thalassemia, where transaminases normalized in 20 and 69% subsequently developed chronic hepatitis during a 8-year follow-up [50]. Unfortunately, there was no testing for HCV RNA and histological assessment was not performed.

Other high-risk populations are cancer survivors, transplant recipients, and hemodialysis patients. On serologic testing of 203 pediatric cancer survivors, 41 (20%) were anti-HCV positive, and of those with chronic liver disease, 50% were positive for anti-HCV [51]. A higher prevalence of HCV infection was seen in children treated for solid tumors compared to leukemia, although the reason for this difference was not clear. Another study where liver biopsy was performed revealed that more severe liver lesions were found in childhood cancer survivors infected with HCV [52]. In the early 1990s the incidence of HCV infection after liver transplantation was reported to be approximately 15% and it was also known that a significant proportion of those previously infected with HCV will reinfect the newly transplanted liver [53]. In a retrospective study, 149 pediatric recipients were evaluated 9 months to 5 years postliver transplant and 14 (9%) were found to be HCV positive [54]. Of the 14, 6 were HCV positive before transplant and reinfected the new liver graft. A delay in antibody seroconversion in this immunosuppressed population was noted, making it difficult to accurately diagnose the cause of graft dysfunction posttransplant. Determination of HCV RNA by PCR is useful as this allows diagnosis of HCV infection before antibody is produced and permits appropriate change in immunosuppression in a timely manner. Similar to prevalence in adult hemodialysis patients, 20% of pediatric hemodialysis patients were found to be HCV positive using first-generation enzyme-linked immunosorbent assay [55].

HCV has also been implicated in "cryptogenic cirrhosis" in adults and children. A study done between 1976 and 1990 showed that 48% of 33 Italian children who had been labeled as having "cryptogenic cirrhosis" had anti-HCV antibodies [56]. While two-thirds had history of parenteral exposure, a third did not. Only 11% of the children achieved biochemical remission over a 5-year follow-up period, leading the authors to conclude that chronic HCV infection, although mildly symptomatic, is associated with a wide range of lesions including cirrhosis and has a low rate of spontaneous remission.

HCV and HIV

In the USA, about 8% of those with chronic HCV infection may be HIV coinfected and conversely, a quarter of HIV-infected individuals in the Western world have chronic HCV infection [11]. The high prevalence of HCV/HIV infection is not unexpected because both viruses are transmitted by the same routes and both are able to evade host immune responses because of a high mutation rate resulting from rapid replication and a lack of "proof-reading" capabilities [57]. Compared to those without HIV, coinfected patients have higher HCV RNA levels and more rapid progression of hepatic fibrosis [58]. Perinatal transmission of HCV is also much higher in coinfected patients. With the advent of highly active antiretroviral treatment, HIV-related mortality has declined, and HCV-related liver disease is a leading cause of hospitalization and death in this population [57].

Conclusion

The incidence of new HCV infections has been declining, but it remains a major cause of chronic liver disease and is the leading cause of liver transplantation in adults in the USA. After universal testing of blood donors for anti-HCV was commenced in 1992, vertical or perinatal transmission has become the most common mode of HCV transmission in children in this country. HCV is a highly heterogeneous pathogen and exists as a quasispecies, with several genotypes and subtypes. The distribution of HCV genotypes reflects the epidemiology of HCV and is also strongly associated with particular routes of transmission. Genotype 1 is most prevalent in the USA. Majority of HCV-infected individuals fail to clear the virus by 6 months and develop chronic hepatitis. A link between HCV and autoimmunity has also been proposed. Natural history data of HCV in pediatrics are sparse and histological correlation has been performed in a small fraction of the affected population. Those coinfected with HIV show higher HCV RNA levels and a more rapid progression to cirrhosis. Future research should explore and identify mechanisms that lead to inadequate immune response after HCV infection, the role of the quasispecies, the relevance of the host genetic factors, and mechanisms of immunosuppression induced by the virus.

References

1. Alter MJ, Kruszon-Moran D, Nainan OV, McQuillan GM, Gao F, Moyer LA et al. The prevalence of hepatitis C virus infection in the United States, 1988 through 1994. N Engl J Med 1999;341(8):556–562.
2. Aach RD, Stevens CE, Hollinger FB, Mosley JW, Peterson DA, Taylor PE et al. Hepatitis C virus infection in post-transfusion hepatitis. An analysis with first- and second-generation assays. N Engl J Med 1991;325(19):1325–1329.
3. Koretz RL, Brezina M, Polito AJ, Quan S, Wilber J, Dinello R et al. Non-A, non-B posttransfusion hepatitis: comparing C and non-C hepatitis. Hepatology 1993;17(3):361–365.
4. Choo QL, Kuo G, Weiner AJ, Overby LR, Bradley DW, Houghton M. Isolation of a cDNA clone derived from a blood-borne non-A, non-B viral hepatitis genome. Science 1989; 244(4902):359–362.
5. Kuo G, Choo QL, Alter HJ, Gitnick GL, Redeker AG, Purcell RH et al. An assay for circulating antibodies to a major etiologic virus of human non-A, non-B hepatitis. Science 1989; 244(4902):362–364.
6. Martell M, Esteban JI, Quer J, Genesca J, Weiner A, Esteban R et al. Hepatitis C virus (HCV) circulates as a population of different but closely related genomes: quasispecies nature of HCV genome distribution. J Virol 1992;66(5):3225–3229.
7. Farci P, Quinti I, Farci S, Alter HJ, Strazzera R, Palomba E et al. Evolution of hepatitis C viral quasispecies and hepatic injury in perinatally infected children followed prospectively. Proc Nat Acad Sci U S A 2006;103(22):8475–8480.
8. Gonzalez-Peralta RP, Qian K, She JY, Davis GL, Ohno T, Mizokami M et al. Clinical implications of viral quasispecies heterogeneity in chronic hepatitis C. J Med Virol 1996;49(3): 242–247.
9. Narkewicz MR, Cabrera R, Gonzalez-Peralta RP. The "C" of viral hepatitis in children. Semin Liver Dis 2007;27(3):295–311.

10. Robertson B, Myers G, Howard C, Brettin T, Bukh J, Gaschen B et al. Classification, nomenclature, and database development for hepatitis C virus (HCV) and related viruses: proposals for standardization. International Committee on Virus Taxonomy. Arch Virol 1998;143(12): 2493–2503.
11. Ghany MG, Strader DB, Thomas DL, Seeff LB. Diagnosis, management, and treatment of hepatitis C: an update. Hepatology 2009;49(4):1335–1374.
12. Armstrong GL, Wasley A, Simard EP, McQuillan GM, Kuhnert WL, Alter MJ. The prevalence of hepatitis C virus infection in the United States, 1999 through 2002. Ann Intern Med 2006;144(10):705–714.
13. Afdhal NH. The natural history of hepatitis C. Semin Liver Dis 2004;24(Suppl 2):3–8.
14. Kim WR, Gross JB, Jr., Poterucha JJ, Locke GR, 3rd, Dickson ER. Outcome of hospital care of liver disease associated with hepatitis C in the United States. Hepatology 2001;33(1):201–206.
15. Tanaka Y, Hanada K, Mizokami M, Yeo AE, Shih JW, Gojobori T et al. Inaugural Article: A comparison of the molecular clock of hepatitis C virus in the United States and Japan predicts that hepatocellular carcinoma incidence in the United States will increase over the next two decades. Proc Nat Acad Sci U S A 2002;99(24):15584–15589.
16. Suchy FJ, Sokol RJ, Balistreri WF, (eds). Liver Disease in Children. 3rd ed. New York: Cambridge University Press, 2007.
17. Zeuzem S, Teuber G, Lee JH, Ruster B, Roth WK. Risk factors for the transmission of hepatitis C. J Hepatol 1996;24(2 Suppl):3–10.
18. Kenny-Walsh E. Clinical outcomes after hepatitis C infection from contaminated anti-D immune globulin. Irish Hepatology Research Group. N Engl J Med 1999;340(16):1228–1233.
19. National Institutes of Health Consensus Development Conference Panel statement management of hepatitis C. Hepatology 1997;26(3 Suppl 1):2S–10S.
20. Guido M, Rugge M, Jara P, Hierro L, Giacchino R, Larrauri J et al. Chronic hepatitis C in children: the pathological and clinical spectrum. Gastroenterology 1998;115(6):1525–1529.
21. Donahue JG, Munoz A, Ness PM, Brown DE, Jr., Yawn DH, McAllister HA, Jr. et al. The declining risk of post-transfusion hepatitis C virus infection. N Engl J Med 1992;327(6): 369–373.
22. Jhaveri R, Grant W, Kauf TL, McHutchison J. The burden of hepatitis C virus infection in children: estimated direct medical costs over a 10-year period. J Pediatr 2006;148(3): 353–358.
23. American Academy of Pediatrics. Committee on Infectious Diseases. Hepatitis C virus infection. Pediatrics 1998;101(3 Pt 1):481–485.
24. Puro V, Girardi E, Ippolito G, Lo-Presti E, Benedetto A, Zaniratti S et al. Prevalence of hepatitis B and C viruses and human immunodeficiency virus infections in women of reproductive age. Br J Obstet Gynaecol 1992;99(7):598–600.
25. Yeung LT, To T, King SM, Roberts EA. Spontaneous clearance of childhood hepatitis C virus infection. J Viral Hepat 2007;14(11):797–805.
26. European Paediatric Hepatitis C Virus Network. Three broad modalities in the natural history of vertically acquired hepatitis C virus infection. Clin Infect Dis 2005;41(1):45–51.
27. Resti M, Jara P, Hierro L, Azzari C, Giacchino R, Zuin G et al. Clinical features and progression of perinatally acquired hepatitis C virus infection. J Med Virol 2003;70(3): 373–377.
28. Jara P, Resti M, Hierro L, Giacchino R, Barbera C, Zancan L et al. Chronic hepatitis C virus infection in childhood: clinical patterns and evolution in 224 white children. Clin Infect Dis 2003;36(3):275–280.
29. D'Souza R, Glynn MJ, Ushiro-Lumb I, Feakins R, Domizio P, Mears L et al. Prevalence of hepatitis C-related cirrhosis in elderly Asian patients infected in childhood. Clin Gastroenterol Hepatol 2005;3(9):910–917.
30. Goodman ZD, Makhlouf HR, Liu L, Balistreri W, Gonzalez-Peralta RP, Haber B et al. Pathology of chronic hepatitis C in children: liver biopsy findings in the Peds-C Trial. Hepatology 2008;47(3):836–843.

31. Mohan P, Colvin C, Glymph C, Chandra RR, Kleiner DE, Patel KM et al. Clinical spectrum and histopathologic features of chronic hepatitis C infection in children. J Pediatr 2007;150(2): 168–174, 174 e161.
32. Dolganiuc A, Szabo G. T cells with regulatory activity in hepatitis C virus infection: what we know and what we don't. J Leuk Biol 2008;84(3):614–622.
33. Bowen DG, Walker CM. Adaptive immune responses in acute and chronic hepatitis C virus infection. Nature 2005;436(7053):946–952.
34. Farci P, Bukh J, Purcell RH. The quasispecies of hepatitis C virus and the host immune response. Springer Semin Immunopathol 1997;19(1):5–26.
35. Weiner A, Erickson AL, Kansopon J, Crawford K, Muchmore E, Hughes AL et al. Persistent hepatitis C virus infection in a chimpanzee is associated with emergence of a cytotoxic T lymphocyte escape variant. Proc Nat Acad Sci U S A 1995;92(7):2755–2759.
36. Tsai SL, Chen YM, Chen MH, Huang CY, Sheen IS, Yeh CT et al. Hepatitis C virus variants circumventing cytotoxic T lymphocyte activity as a mechanism of chronicity. Gastroenterology 1998;115(4):954–965.
37. Grebely J, Thomas DL, Dore GJ. HCV reinfection studies and the door to vaccine development. J Hepatol 2009;51(4):628–631.
38. Gerlach JT, Diepolder HM, Zachoval R, Gruener NH, Jung MC, Ulsenheimer A et al. Acute hepatitis C: high rate of both spontaneous and treatment-induced viral clearance. Gastroenterology 2003;125(1):80–88.
39. Lenzi M, Johnson PJ, McFarlane IG, Ballardini G, Smith HM, McFarlane BM et al. Antibodies to hepatitis C virus in autoimmune liver disease: evidence for geographical heterogeneity. Lancet 1991;338(8762):277–280.
40. Manns MP, Griffin KJ, Sullivan KF, Johnson EF. LKM-1 autoantibodies recognize a short linear sequence in P450IID6, a cytochrome P-450 monooxygenase. J Clin Invest 1991;88(4): 1370–1378.
41. Mackie FD, Peakman M, Yun M, Sallie R, Smith H, Davies ET et al. Primary and secondary liver/kidney microsomal autoantibody response following infection with hepatitis C virus. Gastroenterology 1994;106(6):1672–1675.
42. Vento S, Cainelli F, Renzini C, Concia E. Autoimmune hepatitis type 2 induced by HCV and persisting after viral clearance. Lancet 1997;350(9087):1298–1299.
43. Kerkar N, Choudhuri K, Ma Y, Mahmoud A, Bogdanos DP, Muratori L et al. Cytochrome P4502D6(193-212): a new immunodominant epitope and target of virus/self cross-reactivity in liver kidney microsomal autoantibody type 1-positive liver disease. J Immunol 2003;170(3):1481–1489.
44. Ferri S, Muratori L, Quarneti C, Muratori P, Menichella R, Pappas G et al. Clinical features and effect of antiviral therapy on anti-liver/kidney microsomal antibody type 1 positive chronic hepatitis C. J Hepatol 2009;50(6):1093–1101.
45. Blanchette VS, Vorstman E, Shore A, Wang E, Petric M, Jett BW et al. Hepatitis C infection in children with hemophilia A and B. Blood 1991;78(2):285–289.
46. Romero R, Lavine JE. Viral hepatitis in children. Semin Liver Dis 1994;14(3):289–302.
47. Kanesaki T, Kinoshita S, Tsujino G, Yoshioka K, Ikegami N. Hepatitis C virus infection in children with hemophilia: characterization of antibody response to four different antigens and relationship of antibody response, viremia, and hepatic dysfunction. J Pediatr 1993;123(3): 381–387.
48. Esteban R. Epidemiology of hepatitis C virus infection. J Hepatol 1993;17(Suppl 3):S67–S71.
49. Resti M, Azzari C, Rossi ME, Vullo C, Zammarchi E, Vierucci A. Hepatitis C virus antibodies in a long-term follow-up of beta-thalassaemic children with acute and chronic non-A non-B hepatitis. Eur J Pediatr 1992;151(8):573–576.
50. Lai ME, De Virgilis S, Argiolu F, Farci P, Mazzoleni AP, Lisci V et al. Evaluation of antibodies to hepatitis C virus in a long-term prospective study of posttransfusion hepatitis among thalassemic children: comparison between first- and second-generation assay. J Pediatr Gastroenterol Nutr 1993;16(4):458–464.
51. Fink FM, Hocker-Schulz S, Mor W, Puchhammer-Stockl E, Hofmann H, Zoubek A et al. Association of hepatitis C virus infection with chronic liver disease in paediatric cancer patients. Eur J Pediatr 1993;152(6):490–492.

52. Locasciulli A, Cavalletto D, Pontisso P, Cavalletto L, Scovena E, Uderzo C et al. Hepatitis C virus serum markers and liver disease in children with leukemia during and after chemotherapy. Blood 1993;82(8):2564–2567.
53. Ferrell LD, Wright TL, Roberts J, Ascher N, Lake J. Hepatitis C viral infection in liver transplant recipients. Hepatology 1992;16(4):865–876.
54. Dussaix E, de Paillette L, Laurent-Puig P, Martres P, Lykavieris P, Bernard O et al. Hepatitis C virus infection in pediatric liver transplantation. Transplantation 1993;55(4):795–798.
55. Jonas MM, Zilleruelo GE, LaRue SI, Abitbol C, Strauss J, Lu Y. Hepatitis C infection in a pediatric dialysis population. Pediatrics 1992;89(4 Pt 2):707–709.
56. Bortolotti F, Vajro P, Cadrobbi P, Lepore L, Zancan L, Barbera C et al. Cryptogenic chronic liver disease and hepatitis C virus infection in children. J Hepatol 1992;15(1–2):73–76.
57. Sulkowski MS, Benhamou Y. Therapeutic issues in HIV/HCV-coinfected patients. J Viral Hepat 2007;14(6):371–386.
58. Di Martino V, Rufat P, Boyer N, Renard P, Degos F, Martinot-Peignoux M et al. The influence of human immunodeficiency virus coinfection on chronic hepatitis C in injection drug users: a long-term retrospective cohort study. Hepatology 2001;34(6):1193–1199.

Treatment of Chronic Hepatitis C in Children

Karen F. Murray

Key Concepts

- Effective treatments for children infected with HCV are available.
- Children over the age of 2 years with chronic hepatitis C should be considered for treatment.
- Treatment should be encouraged in children with chronic hepatitis C, without contraindications, especially in those with genotype 2 or 3.
- Treatment for chronic hepatitis C has a number of side effects, and treatment of children should be supervised by those experienced with these medications.
- New medications for the treatment of chronic hepatitis C are currently in development.

Keywords Pediatrics • Hepatitis C • Chronic viral hepatitis • Interferon • Ribavirin • Pegylated-interferon

Background

Since its discovery in 1989 [1], there have been many advancements in the understanding of the hepatitis C virus (HCV), its molecular biology, and the epidemiology, pathogenesis, treatment, and prognosis of individuals chronically infected with this virus. The worldwide prevalence of chronic hepatitis C viral infection (CHC) is estimated at 3%, or 170 million chronically infected individuals. The prevalence varies considerably between geographical regions, with Africa and Southeast Asia having prevalence estimates of 5.3 and 2.1%, respectively, and the USA with a rate estimated at 1.7% [2]. In the USA, however, this relatively low-prevalence rate translates to approximately 7 million adults and 100,000 children infected with HCV [3].

K.F. Murray (✉)
Division of Gastroenterology and Hepatology, Seattle Children's Hospital, 4800 Sand Point Way, NE, PO Box 5371/W-7830, Seattle, WA 98105, USA
e-mail: karen.murray@seattlechildrens.org

M.M. Jonas (ed.), *Viral Hepatitis in Children: Unique Features and Opportunities*, Clinical Gastroenterology, DOI 10.1007/978-1-60761-373-2_5,

Prior to 1992, the predominant mode of exposure for adults was via infected blood products or illicit drug use, and for children, infected blood products. Since 1992, however, with the ability to screen blood products for the virus (blood product HCV infection rate is now estimated to be less than 1/10,000–100,000 units) [4–6], the majority of children acquire the virus via maternal–fetal transmission. Accounting for approximately 60% of HCV infections in children, the maternal–fetal transmission rate is estimated at 4–7% of infants born to mothers with detectable HCV RNA (ribonucleic acid); mothers with a HCV RNA$>10^6$ copies/ml ($>2\times10^5$ IU/ml) are more likely to transmit the infection than mothers with a lower HCV RNA levels [7]. Maternal conditions that are likely to allow for increased HCV replication, such as coinfection with Human Immunodeficiency Virus (HIV), may increase the risk of maternal to infant transmission four- to five-fold [8, 9]. Furthermore, perinatal factors such as prolonged rupture of membranes [≥6 h; odds ratio (OR) 9.3 (95% CI, 1.5–179.7)] and internal fetal scalp electrode monitoring [OR 6.7 (95% CI, 1.1–35.9)] appear to be associated with increased risk of maternal–fetal transmission [10].

The rate of spontaneous HCV clearance may vary depending on the mode of acquisition. In those who acquired the infection via the maternal–fetal route, 0–25% spontaneously clear the HCV infection in the first 2–7 years [11–15]. Although some studies have concluded that children who became HCV infected via transfusion may have higher rates of spontaneous clearance [16], at least one study did not find significant differences in the clearance rates (19%) between these modes of acquisition [17].

Children with CHC are typically asymptomatic or have mild non-specific symptoms [16–18]. Clinical signs of disease are present in approximately 20% of children early in infection, with 10% having hepatomegaly [15], and many with intermittently or persistently elevated alanine or aspartate aminotransferase (ALT, AST) [15–17]. Overall, the degree of hepatitis incurred in the pediatric population compared with that in adults with similar duration of infection, genotype, and HCV RNA levels is less [18]. In a study of 121 children aged 2–16 years, however, 38% had moderate and 3% severe inflammation, five patients had bridging fibrosis and two had cirrhosis. The degree of inflammation correlated with the duration of the infection, and the severity of inflammation and fibrosis correlated with each other [19]. Additionally, this analysis revealed that overweight children had more fibrosis than those who were not overweight. They concluded that "the positive correlation of inflammation with duration of infection and fibrosis and of obesity with fibrosis suggest that children with chronic hepatitis C will be at risk for progressive liver disease as they age and possibly acquire other comorbid risk factors" [19]. Since most children with CHC acquired the infection perinatally, one would expect that they would develop the sequelae of chronic liver disease in the second or third decade of life [20]. In fact, hepatocellular carcinoma has been reported in adolescents [3], and liver transplantation for CHC-related liver disease may be required prior to adulthood [21]. As in adults transplanted for CHC, the outcomes are poor for children who require liver transplantation for CHC (patient and graft survival at 5 years in recipients below the age of 17 years, 71.6 and 55%, respectively) [22].

In addition to the physical impact of CHC on children, there is also potential for psychological impact on both the children and their families. In infected adults, CHC correlates with decreases in cognitive functioning and health-related quality of life (HRQOL) [23]. Children with CHC had worse cognitive functioning than a normative sample, but their behavioral and emotional functioning was comparable. Their caregivers, on the other hand, did experience higher stress and strain on the family system [24].

Given the impact of CHC on children and their families, and the risk of advancing liver disease as the children age, treatment of this infection during childhood has significant potential for advantage. By the same token, the treatment itself may have adverse consequences, similar to or different from those in adults, that must be considered. The remainder of this chapter will discuss the considerations that are necessary when anticipating the treatment of CHC in a child, the currently available treatments, their efficacy and side effects, and potential future treatments.

Diagnosis and Evaluation

Since the vast majority of children infected with HCV are asymptomatic, a high level of suspicion is required to detect individuals with CHC. Any individual who was the recipient of blood products prior to 1992 is at risk and hence should be tested for the viral infection. Similarly, intravenous and intranasal drug users, although uncommon in the pediatric age range, are an at-risk sub-population [25, 26]. Children, however, are exposed perinatally when their mothers are infected, and although the transmission rate is relatively low, testing these children is warranted.

The appropriate test is anti-HCV antibody in serum, via enzyme immunoassay techniques (Fig. 1). The American Academy of Pediatrics recommends that infants born to HCV-infected mothers not be tested for anti-HCV antibody until 18 months of age, as passively acquired maternal antibody may be detectable for up to 18 months [27]. Absence of anti-HCV antibody usually indicates that the individual is not infected; however, antibody may be undetectable in the first weeks after HCV exposure, and in immunocompromised individuals. The presence of antibody, on the other hand, implies HCV exposure, but infection must be verified via the detection of HCV RNA by polymerase chain reaction (PCR) assay. The detection of HCV RNA by PCR is highly sensitive and indicates ongoing viremia. In situations where it is important to know an infant's HCV status prior to 18 months of age, HCV RNA by PCR may be used as early as 1–2 months of age [10, 28]; however, there is a higher specificity of the test at 1 month compared to that at birth (97 vs. 22%) [28], and waiting until 2 months may further increase the specificity of the test [10]. As transient HCV RNA negativity can occur early in infection, it is important to verify any negative tests by repeat analysis 6 months later [29]. Again, some infants who are viremic will have spontaneous resolution of infection during the first few years of life.

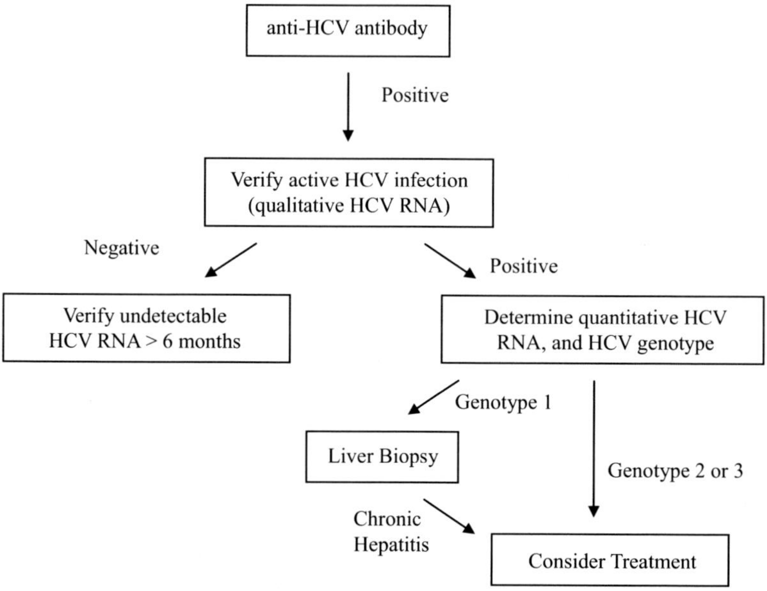

Fig. 1 Evaluation algorithm for consideration of treatment of children with chronic HCV infection

Assessment of hepatic function is advisable at diagnosis of CHC. This can be accomplished by measuring the levels of albumin, bilirubin, and the prothrombin time. A normal ALT in the setting of CHC is not a reliable indicator of the absence of hepatic inflammation, but elevation of ALT is suggestive of hepatic inflammation. Ultrasound interrogation of the liver can verify parenchymal homogeneity and provide evidence of portal hypertension if suspected.

Once the diagnosis of HCV infection is established, secondary evaluations prior to treatment should be undertaken (Table 1). These include genotype (GT) analysis and consideration of liver biopsy for histological evaluation of the infected liver. As discussed in the prior chapter, the HCV genome is a single-stranded, 9.5-kb RNA that encodes a 3,011 amino acid polyprotein. Genomic differences in the RNA by 30–35% of the nucleotide sites characterize different genotypes, of which six have been identified. Genotype 1 (GT1) represents the majority of infections in Western countries, accounting for 67–74% of HCV infections in the US and British populations [30, 31]. GT2 and GT3 represent smaller numbers of infections in the western hemisphere (10–15%), whereas GT4, 5, and 6 are predominant in the Middle East, South Africa, and Southeast Asia, respectively. Within genotypes, closely related subtypes, designated "a" or "b," differing from each other by 20–25% of the nucleotide sites, are further identified. The genotypic identity of the infecting HCV can provide important prognostic information when anticipating treatment, and may dictate different treatment recommendations.

The histological findings might be considered when treatment is being contemplated. Approximately 10–20% of subjects will develop progressive hepatic fibrosis

Table 1 Pretreatment considerations and assessments

History	Laboratory evaluations	Potential contraindications
Psychiatric disease/ depression	HCV RNA PCR	Age < 1 year
Central nervous system disease	HCV genotype	Pregnancy or refusal to practice effective birth control
Retinopathy	AST/ALT	HIV or HBV positive
Sexual activity/birth control	Complete blood count with differential	Poorly controlled depression
Renal disease	Prothrombin time	Anticipated poor compliance with monitoring
Malignancy in the last 5 years	Thyroid function tests	WBC < 3×10^9 l^{-1}; neutrophils < 1.5×10^9 l^{-1}
Thyroid disease	Total IgG and autoantibodies (ASMA, ANA, and ALKMA)	Hgb < 12 g/dl
	HBV and HIV serologies	Platelets < 100×10^9 l^{-1}
	Liver US	Autoantibody positive
	Hepatic histology	Cirrhosis
	Ophthalmologic examination	Recent malignancy
		Renal insufficiency

ASMA anti-smooth muscle antibody, *ANA* anti-neutrophil antibody, *ALKMA* anti-liver–kidney microsomal antibody, *HBV* hepatitis B virus, *HIV* human immunodeficiency antibody, *US* ultrasound, *WBC* white blood cell count, *Hgb* hemoglobin

over 10–20 years of infection. Any individual with non-cirrhotic liver disease should be considered for treatment. Individuals found to have compensated cirrhosis should be considered for treatment only under the monitoring guidance of a transplant center, as treatment is commonly not tolerated and hepatic function may worsen in this setting. Patients with decompensated cirrhosis should be referred for evaluation for transplantation.

Alternatively, the treatment response in those infected with GT2 or GT3 is so good [60–80% sustained virological response (SVR) with pegylated interferon (PEG) plus ribavirin (RV)] that current guidelines support the treatment of these subjects without the need for histological evaluation (Fig. 1).

General Considerations for Treatment

The main goal of therapy in CHC is to achieve sustained eradication of the HCV, defined as SVR (Table 2), undetectable HCV RNA by PCR 24 weeks after the completion of therapy. Secondary, and usually coincident, goals are to halt the progression of the liver disease and to prevent the development of cirrhosis and hepatocellular carcinoma (HCC). Individuals in whom an SVR is achieved enjoy durability of undetectable virus in >99% of cases [32], a condition considered the equivalent to virologic and clinical cure [33].

Table 2 Definitions of virologic response during and after treatment

Terminology	Definition
Rapid virologic response (RVR)	Undetectable HCV RNA (<50 IU/ml) after 4 weeks of treatment
Early virologic response (EVR)	At least a 2 $\log_{10}$ IU/ml decrease in serum HCV RNA from baseline level, after 12 weeks of treatment
End-of-treatment response (ETR)	Undetectable serum HCV RNA (<50 IU/ml) at the end of treatment
Sustained virological response (SVR)	Undetectable serum HCV RNA (<50 IU/ml) 24 weeks after the end of treatment
Non-response	Detectable HCV RNA at 24 weeks of therapy
Relapse	Detection of HCV RNA after an ETR had been achieved

Multiple factors must be considered when counseling a pediatric patient and family about treatment; some are objective, and others more subjective (Table 1). The objective predictors of response to treatment in CHC include HCV RNA levels, HCV genotype, age (> or < 40 years) [34, 35], and potentially body weight/body mass index (BMI). Patients with a quantitative HCV RNA level $<10^6$ copies/ml ($<2\times10^5$ IU/ml) achieve SVR with therapy more frequently than those with an elevated HCV RNA value ($>5\times10^6$ copies/ml) [36]. Similarly, knowledge of the HCV genotype allows for better prediction of treatment response. The SVR rates for GT2 and 3 are 60–80%, respectively, compared to 50% for GT1 [36]. Furthermore, in adults, treatment with PEG plus RV appears to be required for only 6 months for GT2 or GT3, whereas 12 months of therapy is required for GT1 infections [37]. Based on these findings, the pegylated interferon now approved for children (PEG-Intron®, peginterferon alfa-$_{2b}$, Schering–Plough) is approved for 48 weeks of therapy for GT1 and 24 weeks for GT2 and GT3 infections.

The influences of gender and BMI on CHC and the response to treatment are somewhat controversial. In adults, women have milder disease and slower progression compared with men, overall. Confounding variables, such as alcohol consumption, have made this analysis complex, however. Similarly, some authors have found increased treatment response among women compared with men; however, this finding is not consistently observed [35, 38]. The influence of BMI on treatment response has recently been realized, with most studies detecting an improved SVR rate among adults with a BMI < 28 in comparison to that in those with higher BMI [34, 35], but this is not a universal finding [38]. The mechanism by which BMI could influence viral response to therapy is not yet fully understood, although the relative increase in hepatic steatosis with increased BMI and hence increase in insulin resistance could play a significant role in this pathogenesis; it is recognized that hyperinsulinemia is associated with increased GT1-HCV replication [39, 40] and with poorer treatment response [41–43].

Subjective factors should also be considered during treatment deliberations for a child with CHC. The child's and family's QOL, influenced by the social stigmata of harboring a chronic infectious disease, and the family's motivation to "try to eradicate the infection," with knowledge of the treatment and its potential toxicities, must be considered. These considerations in adults extended the treatment recommendations to include those with histologically mild CHC [44]. Although this recommendation was made for individuals over the age of 18 years, pediatric liver specialists generally agree that children meeting the criteria should also be considered for treatment.

The currently approved therapies for CHC include various preparations of interferon-α and ribavirin. Although generally well tolerated in children, these drugs do have a significant number of side effects, and some contraindications should be recognized prior to considering treatment (Table 1). Individuals with compensated or mildly decompensated cirrhosis should be treated only under the monitoring evaluation of a transplant center experienced in pediatric CHC treatment, as the treatment is commonly poorly tolerated under these circumstances, and may worsen the liver function. Severe neurotoxicity in the form of spastic diplegia has been sporadically reported with interferon (IFN)-α treatment of hemangiomas under the age of 1 year [45]. Consequently, the treatment of infants less than 1 year of age should be avoided. Individuals with depression should be closely monitored by mental health professionals familiar with the risk for significant worsening of depression during treatment with IFN, and pre-IFN depression therapy should be considered [46]. Lastly, as the treatment for CHC is associated with minor side effects in approximately 80% of patients, and more severe side effects in 21%, treatment must be closely monitored and pretherapy health status evaluated for any other potential contraindications to treatment. Patients for whom compliance with the treatment and required follow-up are likely to be a challenge should be counseled regarding the requirements prior to embarking on a treatment commitment. Although IFN or ribavirin may be contraindicated in individual health conditions, the risks and benefits to that individual should be considered prior to denying treatment.

Approved Treatments

Interferon-α

Until the mid-1990s IFN-α was the only treatment option for CHC. Type 1 IFNs are naturally occurring proteins produced by leukocytes and are involved in the innate immune response against viruses. When used in the setting of CHC, they are known to inhibit HCV replication, induce cytokine secretion, activate immune cells including natural killer cells and macrophages, and upregulate antigen presentation to T-lymphocytes, thereby increasing the immune recognition of the infection. When used alone, IFN-α resulted in SVR rates of only 10–15% [47]. Although direct comparison of the efficacy of IFN-α monotherapy in children is difficult due to the relative paucity of conclusive controlled trials, a large review of the pediatric

IFN trials to date in 2002, inclusive of 366 treated children, suggested SVR rates of 27% in subjects infected with GT1-HCV and as high as 71% in those infected with GT2 or 3 [48].

Ribavirin

Ribavirin (RV) is a purine nucleoside analog that inhibits the host enzyme inosine monophosphate dehydrogenase and has efficacy against a number of RNA viruses. It also inhibits the HCV polymerase, thereby inhibiting replication of the HCV's genome, inducing mutagenesis, and improving T-lymphocyte response to the infection. Trialed initially as monotherapy, it did not improve the SVR [49], but RV was approved in 1998 to be used in combination with IFN-α where it augmented the SVR to 31–43% [50–52]. Treatment outcome was further optimized by treating for 48 weeks (SVR 38%) rather than for only 24 weeks (SVR 29%) [51]. Subsequent pediatric trials of the combination IFN-α plus RV showed even better results, with an overall SVR of 48%. Again there were genotype differences in response with GT1 subjects exhibiting an SVR of 44% and GT2 and 3 subjects 89% [53–58]. Achieving an SVR predicts durable clearance of HCV in children [59], and adult studies demonstrate lower rates of HCC in subjects who achieved an SVR [60, 61].

The combination of IFN-α_{2b} at a dose of 3 MU/m^2 subcutaneously three times/week, plus ribavirin at a dose of 15 mg/kg/day in two divided doses orally, for 48 weeks was approved by the Federal Drug Administration (FDA) for children aged 3–18 years with CHC [58] (Table 3).

Pegylated-Interferon

The relatively rapid clearance of the IFN from the serum, and differences between the trough and peak concentrations with resultant fluxes in the side effects limit the potential efficacy of this medication. By covalently binding polyethylene glycol to

Table 3 FDA approved therapies for the treatment of children with chronic hepatitis C

Drug	Dose	Dose interval	Route	Duration
IFN	3 MU/m^2	3 times/week	SC	48 weeks
PEG-α_{2b}	60 μg/m^2	Weekly	SC	48 weeks – GT1 24 weeks – GT2 and 3
Ribavirin	15 mg/kg/day	2 divided doses	PO	48 weeks 24 weeks – GT2 and 3[a]

IFN interferon, *PEG-α_{2b}* pegylated interferon-α_{2b}, *SC* subcutaneous injection, *PO* per os, *GT* genotype

[a]When used in combination with PEG-α_{2b}

the IFN molecule, the pharmacodynamics and safety profiles are not substantially altered, yet the differences between the troughs and peaks limited, and the half-life of the medication prolonged. Pegylated-IFN (PEG) is formulated as a 40-kD branched polyethylene molecule bound to IFN-α_{2a} (PEGASYS, Peginterferon alfa-$_{2a}$®, Roche, Ltd), and a linear 12-kD molecule bound to IFN-α_{2b} (PEG-Intron®,Schering Plough); the elimination half-lives of these two preparations is 80 and 40 h, respectively [62]. Although the differences in the two PEG preparations did not result in substantial differences in efficacy when combined with RV [63, 64], the improvement in SVR of PEG/RV compared to IFN/RV therapy was striking. PEG plus RV therapy is now the standard and recommended treatment for adults with CHC, achieving SVR rates of 40–55% in subjects with GT1 infection, and 70–90% for those with GT2 or 3 [65].

The optimal doses of these medications in adults are 180 μg/week for PEG-α_{2a} or 1.5 μg/kg/week for PEG-α_{2b}, subcutaneously. Ribavirin is provided at a dose of 1,000–1,400 mg/day depending on body weight for GT1 and GT4, and 800 mg/day for GT2 and GT3, orally. The recommended duration of therapy has also changed as more controlled trials have accentuated the improved response to therapy of GT2 and GT3 relative to GT1. It is now widely accepted that the appropriate duration of therapy for adults with GT2 or 3 CHC is 6 months (24 weeks), whereas GT1 requires a full year (48 weeks) of therapy [66, 67].

Pediatric experience with PEG and RV treatment is now mounting. In an initial dose-finding study, 6 (43%) of 14 children (age 2–8 years, 13 GT1) given PEG-α_{2a} alone for 48 weeks achieved SVR [68]. Results of several recent uncontrolled trials of PEG/RV treatment of children with CHC have demonstrated SVR rates of 40–53% and 93–100% in those infected with GT1 and 2/3, respectively [68–72]. The importance of RV in the treatment of CHC is underscored by the results of the PEDS-C trial, in which PEG-α_{2a}/RV combination therapy was compared with PEG-α_{2a}/placebo therapy in 114 children aged 5–18 years. In this study, 53% of subjects receiving PEG-α_{2a}/RV achieved SVR compared to only 21% of those who received PEG-α_{2a}/placebo [72]. As discussed earlier, the duration of therapy for adults with CHC is dependent on the HCV genotype, with genotype 2 and 3 requiring only 24 weeks of therapy. Large study comparable information is not yet available on pediatric treatment responses; however, preliminary studies have suggested that genotypes 2 and 3 also require less treatment duration in children [71, 73, 74], and the approved PEG-IFN-α_{2b} (PEG-Intron® Schering-Plough) labeling reflects these findings.

Viral kinetics during treatment may change outcomes, and there are some data to support changes in duration of therapy based on early virologic responses (EVR). EVR (Table 2), even prior to 12 weeks, may allow prediction of SVR, and hence determination of those for whom ongoing therapy is futile. For instance, an EVR at 8 weeks better predicts failure of SVR than analysis at 4 weeks of therapy, but that waiting until 12 weeks of therapy, the current standard EVR for adult treatment, may not be necessary [34]. In pediatrics similar findings are being observed. Viral response analysis during the PEDS-C trial showed that for patients who achieved a RVR, 100% had a SVR. EVR predicted SVR in 94% of the PEG-α_{2a}/RV, and 40%

of the PEG-α_{2a}/placebo-treated subjects [75]. Similarly, Jara et al. [71] demonstrated that 72% of subjects with EVR, but none of the subjects with a less than 2 $\log_{10}$IU/ml drop at 12 weeks, had SVR. In many studies it is observed, however, that some children (7–14%) [71, 72, 75] who do have RNA drop, but not to the magnitude to meet EVR definition, still achieve SVR. SVR is very unlikely in children with detectable RNA after 24 weeks of therapy [68, 69], however, and consequently the current recommendation is to stop therapy if HCV RNA is detectable at 24 weeks.

FDA approval has recently been granted for PEG-α_{2b} subcutaneously at a dose of 60 μg/m^2 once weekly, plus RV (15 mg/kg/day in two divided doses) in children aged 3–18 years, for a full treatment of 48 weeks in GT1 patients, and 24 weeks for GT2 and GT3 (Table 3).

Adverse Events Associated with CHC Treatment

Interferons

In both adults and children, clinical and laboratory adverse effects from interferon therapy are common, and appropriate monitoring is necessary. Quantitative differences in the frequency of adverse effects between IFN and PEG are not substantial, but the weekly administration of the PEG does limit the fluxes in symptoms and generally limits the degree of fever, anorexia, and general flu-like symptoms. In most studies, 100% of subjects will have some adverse effects of the medication, but 80% of these are mild or moderate in severity, and generally fall into the category of "flu-like symptoms" (headache, fever, anorexia, abdominal pain, vomiting, nausea, and myalgias) [58, 71]. Such symptoms usually abate with continuing treatment, and rarely warrant dose change or treatment cessation. Rarely, the interferon dosage will need to be decreased or therapy discontinued if the symptoms become intolerable. More significant adverse events, on the other hand, occur in approximately 20–23% of subjects and include depression, irritability, alopecia, the development of autoantibodies (anti-liver, anti-thyroid), and some laboratory changes [58, 62, 71].

The development of thyroid disease is well described to be associated with both CHC and its treatment with IFN. Although studies report variable rates in children [76], cases of at least transient hypothyroidism are encountered in most large pediatric treatment trials [58, 71, 74]. Monitoring every 3 months for thyroxin and thyroid stimulating hormone levels is advisable, since early identification of thyroid function abnormalities allows appropriate referral and therapy in a timely fashion.

Molecular mimicry between CYP2D6 and the HCV antigens is thought to lead to viral/self-immunological cross-reactivity in some subjects with CHC, leading to expression of anti-liver–kidney microsomal antibody [77, 78]. The presence of this autoantibody appears to be associated with serum aminotransferase flares during interferon therapy, requiring prednisone treatment and potential cessation of the antiviral therapy; however, it is no longer felt to be a contraindication to anti-viral therapy. Furthermore, patients with this autoantibody have similar rates of SVR in comparison to those without the antibody [79]. Pretherapy evaluation for the presence of anti-liver–kidney microsomal antibody and reevaluation in the setting of a hepatitis flare should be considered.

Depression is of more common concern when treating adults, however, and should also be carefully considered and monitored for when treating children. In a large pediatric trial of 118 subjects treated with IFN-α/RV, 13% suffered depression during the study, three of the subjects had suicidal ideation, and one made a suicidal attempt [58]. Any child with a history of depression should be referred for evaluation and ongoing monitoring by a mental health professional during treatment with IFN. A history of suicidal ideation or attempt or untreated major depression should be considered a relative contraindication to treatment.

Anorexia leading to weight loss is encountered in 25–66% of subjects treated with interferons [58, 71]. Similarly, linear growth is impaired during treatment, and both weight and height trend back to baseline after cessation of the therapy. However, full recovery of the lost linear growth has not always been observed, at least in the short term [58, 71]. The PEDS-C group demonstrated that substantial decrements in height, weight, and BMI *z*-scores and % body fat were observed during PEG-α_{2a} therapy. During follow-up, weight, BMI, and fat mass returned to baseline, whereas the height *z*-scores were still lower than baseline 24 and 48 weeks after the cessation of therapy [80].

Severe neurotoxicity in the form of spastic diplegia has been reported in infants treated with IFN-α [45]. Although the mechanism of this neurotoxicity is not understood, the severity of the adverse effect is so significant that treatment of infants younger than 1 year should be avoided, and most pediatric hepatologists avoid the use of this medication in the first 2 years of life. Optic neuritis and retinopathies have also been observed sporadically in subjects treated with IFN-α [81], suggesting the importance of a baseline ophthalmological examination and examinations during therapy as clinically indicated.

The most common laboratory changes encountered with IFN-α or PEG therapy include neutropenia and thrombocytopenia. Serum aminotransferase elevations are less common. Significant neutropenia [absolute neutrophil count (ANC) of 500–1,000 cells/mm^3] occurs in 20–30% of treated individuals, usually within the first month of therapy [58, 71]. Thrombocytopenia is less common, with an acceptable threshold of 100 K/mm^3. As these side effects are dose-dependent, a dose reduction of 20–30% depending on the degree of cellular suppression should be considered, with repeat laboratory analysis (weekly for PEG until stable) suggested (Table 4). Dose adjustment without the need for treatment interruption, in the setting of high compliance is generally not associated with a decrease in SVR. There are no data regarding the use of filgrastim in children who develop neutropenia in association with IFN use, although the rate of serious infection when the ANC is maintained above 500–1,000 cells/mm^3 is low.

Table 4 Recommended laboratory monitoring during HCV therapy

Timing	Test	Interval
During treatment	ALT/AST	Every 1–4 weeks
	CBC with differential	Every 1–4 weeks
	Platelet count	Every 1–4 weeks
	Quantitative HCV RNA	Every 4–12 weeks, then every 12 weeks
	Thyroid function	Every 12 weeks
	Ophthalmologic exam	As clinically indicated
Posttreatment	ALT/AST	4 weeks posttreatment
	CBC with differential	4 weeks posttreatment
	Platelet count	4 weeks posttreatment
	Quantitative HCV RNA	24 weeks posttreatment
	Ophthalmologic exam	24 weeks posttreatment

ALT alanine aminotransferase, *AST* aspartate aminotransferase, *CBC* complete blood count, *HCV RNA* Hepatitis C viral ribonucleic acid

Ribavirin

Although RV is associated with nausea, skin rash, cough, and shortness of breath, the most common side effect is a dose-dependent hemolytic anemia. Approximately 10% of patients experience a 1.4–1.5 g/dl decrease in hemoglobin concentration within the first 4–8 weeks of therapy, with fewer dropping the hemoglobin level to less that 10 g/dl [58, 71, 82]. Dose adjustment is generally only considered for hemoglobin levels below 10 g/dl. The use of exogenous erythropoietin has not been studied in children receiving RV for CHC.

Ribavirin has both teratogenic and embryotoxic effects in animal studies. Although the medication is now known to be important to optimize the SVR after therapy, care must be taken in educating patients of child-bearing age as to the importance of using effective birth control while on this medication and for the 6 months after therapy [83]. Pregnancy testing should be conducted frequently during treatment of adolescents of child-bearing potential.

Treatment of Non-Responders and Those Who Relapse

There are no pediatric studies specifically evaluating the efficacy of retreating patients who either did not respond (detectable HCV RNA at 24 weeks) or relapsed (ETR (end-of-treatment response) but not SVR, Table 2) after initial treatment. Adults retreated with PEG/RV after prior non-response to IFN or PEG/RV achieve SVR rates of 40 and 10%, respectively [84, 85]. Fifty percent of adults who relapsed after IFN monotherapy then retreated with PEG/RV achieve SVR, and those with GT 2 or 3 have a higher rate of success [84–86].

Small pediatric trials of non-responder patients suggest that similar results may be seen with retreatment in children. Six of nine children who were unresponsive to IFN secured SVR upon retreatment with IFN/RV [54]. Six of 12 patients previously unresponsive to IFN/RV achieved ETR (SVR was not reported) with PEG/RV [87] and two of five patients retreated with PEG/RV after non-response to IFN achieved SVR [69].

Treatment of Special Pediatric Populations

Patients with Thalassemia

Due to the risk of hemolysis with the use of ribavirin, it has been considered contraindicated to use this medication in patients with hemolytic conditions such as thalassemia. Children who received transfusion of blood products prior to 1992 are at risk of having contracted HCV, and in Asia the prevalence of HCV in patients with thalassemia varies from 20 to 64% [88–90]. These children are usually infected in the first decade of life, and in the setting of iron-overload and the associated immune deficiencies, are prone to develop CHC. Additionally, there is concern that the HCV and iron-overload could act synergistically in the development of cirrhosis and HCC. Monotherapy with IFN in transfusion-dependent β-thalassemic children results in SVR in 58.7–87.5% [90, 91]. At a cost of only slightly increased transfusion rates combination therapy with PEG/RV may also prove to be possible [92, 93].

Patients with Viral Coinfections

There is little information regarding coinfected children; however, there appears to be mutual inhibition of viral replication in adults who are coinfected with HCV and hepatitis B virus (HBV). In HBV/HCV-infected adults, the currently preferred therapy is PEG/RV, with efficacy of the PEG against the HBV also realized. HIV/HCV coinfection is a bit more complicated in that HIV accelerates the natural history of HCV. Restoration of immune function and its maintenance via highly active antiretroviral therapy (HAART) reduce the impact of HIV on HCV, but even in this situation, the HCV SVR following PEG/RV appears to be 15–50% lower than that in HCV only infected individuals [94, 95]. Given the lower HCV-treatment response rates in this coinfected population, treatment for 48 weeks is recommended regardless of the GT. Similar recommendations for coinfected children have been made [96].

Transplantation

Adult patients with CHC who undergo solid organ transplantation have persistent HCV viremia and progressive liver disease posttransplant. After liver transplantation for CHC, graft reinfection is nearly universal and approximately 30% will develop cirrhosis or die due to HCV by the fifth posttransplant year. In one study of 67 children who underwent liver transplantation for HCV, the patient and graft survival rates were 71.6% and 55%, respectively, at 5 years [22]. Treatment in these subjects should be initiated with caution and only by those experienced in treating posttransplant patients, due to the risks of intolerance, graft rejection, and mortality [97, 98]. In those who are able to successfully complete treatment, the SVR rates are reasonable. Trials of PEG/RV treatment postliver transplantation in adults show SVRs of 14–45%, with 48 weeks of therapy recommended regardless of HCV genotype [99].

Treatment prior to renal transplantation is recommended for adults with HCV-related renal disease, and treatment for HCV-liver disease is not recommended in the renal transplant patient unless they develop fibrosing cholestatic hepatitis. Treatment of patients with other solid organ transplantation should be made on an individual basis [67].

Treatments in Development

Although PEG/RV provides improved rates of SVR compared with the original IFN monotherapy, SVR rates are still suboptimal in the majority of patients. The goals of therapies in development include better tolerance profiles and improved efficacy. Newer IFN (albumin-IFN) and ribavirin (taribavirin) molecules and specific targeted antiviral therapy for HCV (STAT-C, Specifically Targeted Antiviral Therapy for hepatitis C), targeted to specific steps in the replication cycle of the virus, are currently under investigation. STAT-C potential therapy targets include the NS3 serine protease, NS3 helicase, and NS5B RNA-dependent RNA polymerase.

Albuferon (albumin-IFN-α_{2b}) is a recombinant single polypeptide coded by the fusion of the human IFN-α and serum albumin genes. This has the potential advantage of delayed clearance and hence dosing every 2–4 weeks [62, 100]. *Consensus-IFN* [101, 102], a recombinant type 1 IFN, or *alfacon-1* [103], a completely synthetic IFN, appears to have 5–10 times the biological activity of the current IFNs [62], but it does not yet appear that these drugs have improved efficacy over PEG [104].

Among the STAT-C medications, two protease inhibitors, telaprevir and boceprevir, entered phase III trials in adults in 2008 [105]. Recent PROVE1 and PROVE2 studies of telaprevir/PEG/RV in GT1 infected adults have provided exciting results. Treatment-naïve subjects were treated with triple therapy including telaprevir for the initial 12 weeks and PEG-α_2/RV for 24 weeks. The SVRs were 61 and 69% compared with 41 and 46% with PEG/RV alone for 48 weeks, respectively. There were also far more frequent RVRs (81 vs. 11% – PROBE1, and 69 vs. 13% – PROBE2) which, as found with current therapies, were associated with higher SVR rates [106, 107]. One of the most common side effects with telaprevir is a drug-induced rash that occurs between 8 and 88 days into therapy, and pruritus was a common indication for discontinuation of the drug, being severe in 5% of subjects [106, 107]. Initial results of a similar study (SPRINT1) of boceprevir in combination with PEG-α_2 and RV in treatment-naïve GT1-infected adults demonstrated HCV RNA undetectability in 55–57% of subjects at follow-up week 12 [108]. These drugs have not been tested in children.

The NS5B-encoded RNA-dependent RNA polymerase has active catalytic sites that could be bound by nucleoside analogs, and non-nucleoside polymerase inhibitors could bind at outside sites, providing other potential drug options [105]. Such potential compounds are currently in phase I and II trials. Although a few of these drugs are showing high potency (R1626 and R7128), some have already been withdrawn due to safety concerns [66].

Taribavirin hydrochloride is a liver-targeting pro-drug of RV that is found to release RV primarily at the hepatocyte, without accumulation in erythrocytes. Safety and efficacy improvements of this compound over RV have not yet been illustrated, however [109].

Among the potentially most exciting of the drugs in development are drugs that stimulate the host's immune response against the virus. In CHC, the innate and adaptive immune responses are somewhat dysfunctional. Stimulation of Toll-like receptors (TLR), which are pathogen recognition molecules expressed on immunologic cells, would enhance the ability of the immunologic cells to sense the presence of the HCV and initiate the innate immune response [62, 66, 110]. Current drugs under development include CPG 10101 or Actilon, with agonistic activity with TLR9, and ANA245 or isatoribine, with activity with TLR7 [62, 66, 110].

Summary

Chronic hepatitis C is one of the most common chronic liver diseases in the USA. A high index of suspicion is required for diagnosis given the high percentage of infected individuals who are asymptomatic, especially among children. Despite the wellness of most individuals, progression of HCV-induced liver disease occurs during childhood, potentially influencing the individual's health in the first few decades of life. Treatments are now approved for both adults and children with improved efficacy such that the treatment of most individuals should be considered. Although generally well tolerated, the treatments do carry potentially serious toxicities, and hence treatment should be closely monitored by practitioners experienced with CHC treatment in children. Children under the age of 2 years should not be treated. Although both treatments are approved, PEG/RV is superior to IFN/RV in its frequency of administration, tolerance, and anti-viral efficacy. GT2- and GT3-infected subjects can be successfully treated with just 24 weeks of treatment rather than the 48 weeks required for GT1. Newer therapies are currently under investigation.

References

1. Choo QL, Kuo G, Weinder AJ, Overby LR, Bradley DW, Houghton M. Isolation of a cDNA clone derived from a blood-borne non-A non-B viral hepatitis-genome. Science 1989;244:359–362.
2. Sy T, Jamal MM. Epidemiology of hepatitis C viral infection. Int J Med Sci 2006;3(2):41–46.
3. González-Peralta RP, Langham Jr MR, Andres JM, et al. Hepatocellular carcinoma in 2 young adolescents with chronic hepatitis C. J Pediatr Gastroenterol Nutr 2009;48(5):630–635.
4. Lam NP. Hepatitis C: natural history, diagnosis, and management. Am J Health Syst Pharm 1999;56:961–973.
5. Layden TJ, Lam NP, Wiley TE. Hepatitis C viral dynamics. Clin Liver Dis 1999;3:793–810.
6. Luban NL, Colvin CA, Mohan P, Alter HJ. The epidemiology of transfusion-associated hepatitis C in a children's hospital. Transfusion 2007;47:615–620.
7. Roberts EA, Yeung L. Maternal–infant transmission of hepatitis C virus infection. Hepatology 2002;36:S106–S113.
8. Airoldi J, Berghella V. Hepatitis C and pregnancy. Obstet Gynecol Surv 2006;61:666–672.
9. Airoldi J. Hepatitis C and pregnancy. Obstet Gynecol Surv 2006;61(10):666–672.
10. Mast EE, Hwang L-Y, Seto DSY, et al. Risk factors for perinatal transmission of hepatitis C virus (HCV) and the natural history of HCV infection acquired in infancy. J Infect Dis 2005;192:1880–1889.
11. Tovo P-A, Pembrey LJ, Newell M-L. Persistence rate and progression of vertically acquired hepatitis C infection. J Infect Dis 2000;181:419–424.
12. Yeung LT, To T, King SM, Roberts EA. Spontaneous clearance of childhood hepatitis C virus infection. J Viral Hepat 2007;14(11):797–805.
13. Bortolotti F, Resti M, Giacchino R, et al. Hepatitis C virus infection and related liver disease in children of mothers with antibodies to the virus. J Pediatr 1997;130(6):859–861.
14. Resti M, Jara P, Hierro L, et al. Clinical features and progression of perinatally acquired hepatitis C virus infection. J Med Virol 2003;70(3):373–377.
15. European Pediatric Hepatitis C Virus Network. Three broad modalities in the natural history of vertically acquired hepatitis C virus infection. Clin Infect Dis 2005;41:45–51.
16. Davison SM, Mieli-Vergani G, Kelly DA. Perinatal hepatitis C virus infection: diagnosis and management. Arch Dis Child 2006;91:781–785.
17. Shiraki K, Ohto H, Inaba N, et al. Guidelines for care of pregnant women carrying hepatitis C virus and their infants. Pediatr Int 2008;50(1):138–140.
18. Murray KF, Finn LS, Taylor SL, Seidel KD, Larson AM. Liver histology and alanine amino transferase levels in children and adults with chronic hepatitis C infection. J Pediatr Gastroenterol Nutr 2005;41(5):634–638.
19. Goodman ZD, Makhlouf HR, Liu L, et al. Pathology of chronic hepatitis C in children: liver biopsy findings in the Peds-C Trial. Hepatology 2008;47:836–843.
20. Yeung LT, King SM, Roberts EA. Mother-to-infant transmission of hepatitis C virus. Hepatology 2001;34:223–229.
21. Mohan P, Colvin CA, Glymph C, et al. Clinical spectrum and histopathologic features of chronic hepatitis C infection in children. J Pediatr 2007;150(2):168–174.
22. Barshes NR, Udell IW, Lee TC, et al. The natural history of hepatitis C virus in pediatric liver transplant recipients. Liver Transpl 2006;12(7):1119–1123.
23. Spiegel BM, Younossi ZM, Hays RD, Revicki D, Robbins S, Kanwal F. Impact of hepatitis C on health related quality of life: a systematic review and quantitative assessment. Hepatology 2005;41:790–800.
24. Rodrigue JR, Balistreri W, Haber B, et al. Impact of hepatitis C virus infection on children and their caregivers: quality of life, cognitive, and emotional outcomes. J Pediatr Gastroenterol Nutr 2009;48:341–347.
25. Murray KF, Richardson LP, Morishima C, Owens JWM, Gretch DR. Prevalence of hepatitis C virus infection and risk factors in an incarcerated juvenile population: a pilot study. Pediatrics 2003;111(1):153–157.

26. Garfein RS, Doherty MC, Monterroso ER, Thomas DL, Nelson KE, Vlahov D. Prevalence and incidence of hepatitis C Virus infection among young adult injection drug users. J Acquir Immune Defic Syndr Hum Retrovirol 1998;18(Suppl. 1):S11–S19.
27. American Academy of Pediatrics. Hepatitis C. In: Pickering LK, Baker CJ, Long SS, McMillan JA, eds. Red Book: 2006 report of the Committee on Infectious Diseases, 27th ed. Elk Grove Village, IL: American Academy of Pediatrics, 2006:355–359.
28. Dunn DT, Gibb GM, Healy M, et al. Timing and interpretation of tests for diagnosing perinatally acquired hepatitis C virus infection. Pediatr Infect Dis J 2001;20:715–716.
29. Davison SM, Kelley DA. Management strategies for hepatitis C virus infection in children. Pediatr Drugs 2008;10(6):357–365.
30. Gerner P, Wirth S, Wintermeyer P, Walz A, Jenke A. Prevalence of hepatitis C virus infection in children admitted to an urban hospital. J Infect Dis 2006;52:305–308.
31. Alter MJ, Kruszon-Moran D, Nainan OV, et al. The prevalence of hepatitis C infection in the United States, 1988 through 1994. N Engl J Med 1999;341:556–562.
32. Nelson DR, Davis GL, Jacobson IM, et al. Hepatitis C virus: a critical appraisal of approaches to therapy. Clin Gastroenterol Hepatol 2009;7(4):397–414.
33. National Institute of Health. National Institute of Health consensus development conference statement: management of hepatitis C: 2002. Hepatology 2002;36:S3–S20.
34. Lukasiewicz E, Gorfine M, Freedman LS, et al. Prediction of nonSVR to therapy with pegylated interferon-alpha2a and ribavirin in chronic hepatitis C genotype 1 patients after 4, 8 and 12 weeks of treatment. J Viral Hepat 2010;17(5):345–351.
35. Dahlan Y, Ather HM, Al-ahmadi M, Batwa F, Al-hamoudi W. Sustained virological response in a predominantly hepatitis C virus genotype 4 infected population. World J Gastroenterol 2009;15(35):4429–4433.
36. Ferenci P, Fried MW, Shiffman ML, et al. Predicting sustained virological responses in chronic hepatitis C patients treated with peginterferon alfa-2a (40 KD)/ribavirin. J Hepatol 2005;43:425–433.
37. Rizzetto M. Treatment of hepatitis C virus genotype 2 or 3 with pegylated interferon plus ribavirin. J Hepatol 2004;42:275–278.
38. Husa P, Slesinger P, Stroblová H, Svobodník A. The effect of patient's body weight, gender and baseline viral load on the efficacy of hepatitis C therapy. Vnitr Lek 2006;52(6): 590–595.
39. Harrison SA. Correlation between insulin resistance and hepatitis C viral load. Hepatology 2006;43:1168–1169.
40. Moucari R, Asselah T, Cazals-Hatem D, et al. Insulin resistance in chronic hepatitis C: association with genotype 1 and 4, serum HCV RNA level, and liver fibrosis. Gastroenterology 2008;134:416–423.
41. Delgado-Borrego A, Healey D, Negre B, et al. Influence of body mass index on outcome of pediatric chronic hepatitis C virus infection. J Pediatr Gastroenterol Nutr. 2010 Jun 3. PMID: 20531022.
42. Grasso A, Malfatti F, De Leo P, et al. Insulin resistance predicts rapid virological response in non-diabetic, non-cirrhotic genotype 1 HCV patients treated with peginterferon alpha-2b plus ribavirin. J Hepatol 2009;51(6):984–990. DOI:10.1016/j.hep.2009.07.008.
43. Romero-Gomez M, Del Mar Viloria M, Andrade RJ, et al. Insulin resistance impairs sustained response rate to peginterferon plus ribavirin in chronic hepatitis C patients. Gastroenterology 2005;128:636–641.
44. National Institute for Health and Clinical Excellence. Peginterferon alfa and ribavirin for the treatment of mild chronic hepatitis C. London: NICE, 2006 (accessed at http://guidance.nice.org.uk/TA106/Guidance).
45. Wörle H, Maass E, Köhler B, Treuner J. Interferon alpha-2a therapy in haemangiomas of infancy: spastic diplegia as a severe complication. Eur J Pediatr 1999;158(4):344.
46. Sockalingam S, Abbey SE. Managing depression during hepatitis C treatment. Can J Psychiatry 2009;54(9):614–625.
47. Davis GL. Treatment of acute and chronic hepatitis C. Clin Liver Dis 1997;1:615–630.

48. Jacobson KR, Murray K, Zellos A, Schwarz KB. An analysis of published trials of Interferon monotherapy in children with chronic hepatitis C. J Pediatr Gastroenterol Nutr 2002; 34(1):52–58.
49. Querenghi F, Yu Q, Billaud G, Maertens G, Trepo C, Zoulim F. Evolution of hepatitis C virus genome in chronically infected patients receiving ribavirin monotherapy. J Viral Hepat 2001;8:120–131.
50. Reichard O, Norkrans G, Fryden A, Braconier JH, Sonnerborg A, Weiland O. Randomized, double-blind, placebo-controlled trial of interferon alpha-2b with and without ribavirin for chronic hepatitis C: The Swedish Study Group. Lancet 1998;351:83–87.
51. Poynard T, Marcellin P, Lee S, et al. Randomised trial of interferon alpha2b plus ribavirin for 48 weeks or for 24 weeks versus interferon alpha2b plus placebo for 48 weeks for treatment of chronic infection with hepatitis C virus. International Hepatitis Interventional Therapy Group (IHIT). Lancet 1998;352:1426–1432.
52. McHutchison JG, Gordon SC, Schiff ER, et al. Interferon alfa-2b alone or in combination with ribavirin as initial treatment for chronic hepatitis C. N Engl J Med 1998; 339(21):1485–1492.
53. Suoglu DOD, Elkabes B, Sokueu S, Saner G. Does interferon and ribavirin combination therapy increase the rate of treatment response in children with hepatitis C. J Pediatr Gastroenterol Nutr 2002;34(2):199–206.
54. Wirth S, Lang T, Gehring S, Gerner P. Recombinant alfa-interferon plus ribavirin therapy in children and adolescents with chronic hepatitis C. Hepatology 2002;36:1280–1284.
55. Hartman C, Berkowitz D, Rimon N, Shamir R. The effect of early treatment in children with chronic hepatitis. J Pediatr Gastroenterol Nutr 2003;37:252–257.
56. Figlerowicz M, Sluzewski W, Kowala-Piaskowska A, Mozer-Lizewska I. Interferon alpha and ribavirin in the treatment of children with chronic hepatitis C. Eur J Pediatr 2004; 1633:265–267.
57. Lackner H, Moser A, Deutsch J, et al. Interferon-alpha and ribavirin in treating children and young adults with chronic hepatitis C after malignancy. Pediatrics 2000;106(4):E53.
58. González-Peralta RP, Deirdre KA, Haber B, et al. Interferon alfa-2b with ribavirin for children with chronic hepatitis C: efficacy, safety, and pharmacokinetics. Hepatology 2005;42: 1010–1018.
59. Kelly D, Haber B, Gonzalez-Peralta RP, et al. Sustained virologic response to interferon alfa-2b plus ribavirin predicts long-term clearance of HCV in pediatric patients at 5 year follow-up. J Hepatol 2008;48(Suppl. 2):S298.
60. Nishiguchi S, Kuroki T, Nakatani S. Randomised trial of effects of interferon on the incidence of hepatocellular carcinoma in chronic active hepatitis C with cirrhosis. Lancet 1995; 346:1051–1055.
61. Nishiguchi S, Shiomi S, Nakatani S, et al. Prevention of hepatocellular carcinoma in patients with chronic active hepatitis C and cirrhosis. Lancet 2001;357(9251):196–197.
62. Karnsakul W, Alford MK, Schwarz KB. Managing pediatric hepatitis C: current and emerging treatment options. Ther Clin Risk Manag 2009;5:651–660.
63. Di Bisceglie AM, Ghalib RH, Hamzeh FM, Rustgi VK. Early virologic response after peginterferon alpha-2a plus ribavirin or peginterferon alpha-2b plus ribavirin treatment in patients with chronic hepatitis C. J Viral Hepat 2007;14:721–729.
64. Yenice N, Mehtap O, Gumrah M, Arican N. The efficacy of pegylated interferon alpha 2a or 2b plus ribavirin in chronic hepatitis C patients. Turk J Gastroenterol 2006;17:94–98.
65. Dalgard O, Bjøro K, Ring-Larsen H, et al. Pegylated interferon alfa and ribavirin for 14 vs 24 weeks in patients with hepatitis C virus genotype 2 or 3 and rapid virological response. Hepatology 2008;47(1):35–42.
66. Deutsch M, Hadziyannis SJ. Old and emerging therapies in chronic hepatitis C: an update. J Viral Hepat 2008;15:2–11.
67. Ghany MG, Strader DB, Thomas DL, Seeff LB. Diagnosis, management, and treatment of hepatitis C: an update. Hepatology 2009;49(4):1337–1374.

68. Schwarz KB, Mohan P, Narkewicz M, et al. Safety, efficacy and pharmacokinetics of peginterferon alpha-2a (40KD) in children with chronic hepatitis C. J Pediatr Gastroenterol Nutr 2006;4:499–505.
69. Wirth S, Pieper-Boustani H, Lang T, et al. Peginterferon alfa-2b plus ribavirin treatment in children and adolescents with chronic hepatitis C. Hepatology 2005;41(5):1013–1018.
70. Wirth S, Ribes-Koninckx C, Bortolotti F, et al. Children with HCV infection show high sustained virologic response rates on peginterferon alfa-2b plus ribavirin treatment. Hepatology 2008;48:392A (abstract).
71. Jara P, Hierro L, de la Vega A, et al. Efficacy and safety of peginterferon alfa2b and ribavirin combination therapy in children with chronic hepatitis C infection. Pediatr Infect Dis J 2008;27:142–148.
72. Schwarz KB, González-Peralta RP, Murray KF, et al. Peginterferon with or without ribavirin for chronic hepatitis C in children and adolescents: final results of the PEDS-C trial. Hepatology 2008;48:418A (abstract).
73. Sokal E, Bourgois A, Stephenne X, et al. Multicenter trial of peg-interferon α2a and ribavirin in pediatric chronic hepatitis C. Hepatology 2009;50(4 Suppl.):418A.
74. Murray KF, Rodrigue JR, Gonzalez-Peralta RP, et al. Design of the PEDS-C trial: pegylated interferon +/− ribavirin for children with chronic hepatitis C viral infection. Clin Trials 2007; 4(6):661–673.
75. Schwarz KB, Valsamakis A, Balistreri W, et al. Early changes in viral load predict sustained viral response (SVR) in the PEDS-C trial. Hepatology 2009;50(4 Suppl.):419A.
76. Tomer Y, Menconi F. Interferon induced thyroiditis. Best Pract Res Clin Endocrinol Metab 2009;23(6):703–712.
77. Marceau G, Lapierre P, Beland K, Soudeyns H, Alverez F. LKM1 autoantibodies in chronic hepatitis C infection: a case of molecular mimicry? Hepatology 2005;42:675–682.
78. Yamamoto AM, Cresteil D, Boniface O, Clerc FF, Alverez F. Identification and analysis of cytochrome P459IId6 antigenic sites recognized by anti-liver–kidney microsome type-1 antibodies (LKM 1). Eur J Immunol 1993;23:1105–1111.
79. Ferri S, Muratori L, Quarneti C, et al. Clinical features and effect of antiviral therapy on anti-liver/kidney microsomal antibody type 1 positive chronic hepatitis C. J Hepatol 2009;50:1093–1101.
80. Jonas MM, Balistreri W, Gonzalez-Peralta RP, et al. Changes in body mass index and body composition in children treated with peginterferon for chronic hepatitis C in the PEDS-C trial. Hepatology 2009;50(4 Suppl.):636A.
81. Panetta JD, Gilani N. Interferon-induced retinopathy and its risk in patients with diabetes and hypertension undergoing treatment for chronic hepatitis C virus infection. Aliment Pharmacol Ther 2009;30(6):597–602.
82. Jonas MM. Children with hepatitis C. Hepatology 2002;36:S173–S178.
83. Krilov LR. Safety issues related to the administration of ribavirin. Pediatr Infect Dis J 2002;21:479–481.
84. Shiffmann ML, Di Bisceglie AM, Lindsay KL, et al. Peginterferon alfa-2a and ribavirin in patients with chronic hepatitis C who failed prior treatment. Gastroenterology 2004;126: 1015–1023.
85. Jacobsen IM, Ahmed F, Russo MW, et al. Pegylated interferon alfa-2b plus ribavirin in patients with chronic hepatitis C: a trial in non-responders to interferon monotherapy or combination therapy and in combination therapy relapsers: final results. Gastroenterology 2003;124:A540.
86. Davis GL, Esteban-Mur R, Rustgi V, et al. Interferon alfa-2b alone or in combination with ribavirin for the treatment of relapse of chronic hepatitis C. N Engl J Med 1998;339(21): 1493–1499.
87. Pawlowska M, Palewicz E, Halota W. Early virologic response in retherapy with pegylated interferon alpha 2b plus ribavirin in children with chronic hepatitis C. Przegl Epidemiol 2006;60(1):71–77.

88. Wanachiwanawin W, Luengrojanakul P, Sirangkapracha P, Leowattana W, Fucharoen S. Prevalence and clinical significance of hepatitis C virus infection in Thai patients with thalassemia. Int J Hematol 2003;78:374–378.
89. Ansar MM, Koolobandi A. Prevalence of hepatitis C virus infection in thalassemia and haemodialysis patients in north Iran-Rasht. J Viral Hepat 2002;9:390–392.
90. Mohan N, Majumdar I, Kaul D, et al. Prevalence of hepatitis C infection and response of treatment to interferon alpha in beta thalassemia patients. J Pediatr Gastroenterol Nutr 2004;39(Suppl. 1):S174.
91. Di Marco V, Lo Iacono O, Almasio P, et al. Long term efficacy of alpha-interferon in beta-thalassemics with chronic hepatitis C. Blood 1997;90(6):2207–2212.
92. Harmatz P, Jonas MM, Kwiatkowski JL, et al. Safety and efficacy of pegylated interferon α-2a and ribavirin for the treatment of hepatitis C in patients with thalassemia. Haematologica 2008;93:1247–1251.
93. Mohan N, Ganeja V, Kaul D, Khanna V, et al. PEG interferon alpha 2A (40KD) plus ribavirin treatment in thalassemic children and adolescents with chronic hepatitis C. J Pediatr Gastroenterol Nutr 2007;44(Suppl. 1):e-144 (abstract).
94. Tural C, Galeras JA, Planas R, et al. Differences in virological response to pegylated interferon and ribavirin between hepatitis C virus (HCV)-monoinfected and HCV–HIV-coinfected patients. Antivir Ther 2008;13(8):1047–1055.
95. Asian Pacific Association for the Study of the Liver (APASL) Hepatitis C Working Party, McCaughan GW, Omata M, et al. Asian Pacific Association for the Study of the Liver consensus statements on the diagnosis, management and treatment of hepatitis C virus infection. J Gastroenterol Hepatol 2007;22(5):615–633.
96. Mofenson LM, Brady MT, Danner SP, et al. Guidelines for the prevention and treatment of opportunistic infections among HIV-exposed and HIV-infected children: recommendations from CDC, the National Institutes of Health, the HIV Medicine Association of the Infectious Diseases Society of America, the Pediatric Infectious Diseases Society, and the American Academy of Pediatrics. MMWR Recomm Rep 2009;58(RR-11):1–166.
97. Pereira BJ, Natov SN, Bouthot BA, et al. Effects of hepatitis C infection and renal transplantation on survival in end-stage renal disease. The New England Organ Bank Hepatitis C Study Group. Kidney Int 1998;53:1374–1381.
98. Wright TL, Donegan E, Hsu HH, et al. Recurrent and acquired hepatitis C viral infection in liver transplant recipients. Gastroenterology 1992;103:317–322.
99. Watt K, Veldt B, Charlton M. A practical guide to the management of HCV infection following liver transplantation. Am J Transplant 2009;9:1–7.
100. Osborn BL, Olsen HS, Nardelli B, et al. Pharmacokinetic and pharmacodynamic studies of a human serum albumin-interferon-alpha fusion protein in cynomolgus monkeys. J Pharmacol Exp Ther 2002;303:540–548.
101. Heathcote EJ, Keeffe EB, Lee SS, et al. Re-treatment of chronic hepatitis C with consensus interferon. Hepatology 1998;27:1136–1143.
102. Moskovitz DN, Manoharan P, Heathcote EJ. High dose consensus interferon in nonresponders to interferon alpha-2b and ribavirin with chronic hepatitis C. Can J Gastroenterol 2003;17:479–482.
103. Melian EB, Plosker GL. Interferon alfacon-1: a review of its pharmacology and therapeutic efficacy in the treatment of chronic hepatitis C. Drugs 2001;61:1661–1691.
104. Bacon BR, Shiffman ML, Mendes F, et al. Retreating chronic hepatitis C with daily interferon alfacon-1/ribavirin after nonresponse to pegylated interferon/ribavirin: DIRECT results. Hepatology 2009;49(6):1838–1846.
105. Brown NA. Progress towards improving antiviral therapy for hepatitis C with hepatitis C virus polymerase inhibitors. Part 1. Nucleoside analogues. Expert Opin Investig Drugs 2009;18:709–725.
106. Hezode C, Forestier N, Dushieko G, et al. PROVE2 Study. Telaprevir with peginterferon with or without ribavirin for chronic HCV infection. N Engl J Med 2009;360:1839–1850.

107. McHutchison JG, Everson GT, Gordon SC, et al. PROVE1 Study. Telaprevir with peginterferon and ribavirin for chronic HCV genotype 1 infection. N Engl J Med 2009;360:1827–1838.
108. Kwo P, Lawitz EJ, McCone J, et al. HCV SPRINT-1: boceprevir plus peginterferon alfa-2b/ribavirin for treatment of genotype 1 chronic hepatitis C in previously untreated patients. Hepatology 2008;48:268A (abstract).
109. Schiff ER. Emerging strategies for pegylated interferon combination therapy. Nat Clin Pract Gastroenterol Hepatol 2007;4(Suppl. 1):S17–S21.
110. Horsmans Y, Berg T, Desager JP, et al. Isatoribine, an agonist of TLR7, reduces plasma virus concentration in chronic hepatitis C infection. Hepatology 2005;42:724–731.

Hepatitis D and Hepatitis E in Children

Rima Fawaz

Key Concepts

- Hepatitis D virus is a defective virus whose replication depends on an obligatory simultaneous infection with hepatitis B virus.
- Hepatitis D virus has a worldwide but non-uniform distribution.
- The clinical presentation of hepatitis D varies from asymptomatic infection to, more typically, severe icteric hepatitis.
- Chronic hepatitis D is associated with rapid progression to cirrhosis and increased risk of hepatocellular carcinoma.
- There is no effective therapy for HDV infection. Universal vaccination for hepatitis B is key to prevention of chronic hepatitis D.
- Hepatitis E is transmitted predominantly by the fecal-oral route
- The clinical presentation of acute hepatitis E is similar to that of other forms of viral hepatitis; hence the diagnosis needs to be suspected in the appropriate clinical context.
- Hepatitis E therapy is supportive; HEV vaccines are being developed.

Keywords HDV • Hepatitis delta • Virology • Epidemiology • Pathogenesis • Clinical manifestations • Diagnosis • Treatment • HEV • Child

Hepatitis D

Hepatitis D, also known as delta hepatitis, is caused by a defective RNA virus. In 1977, Rizzetto and associates reported a nuclear antigen, "delta antigen," in hepatocytes of patients with chronic hepatitis B [1]. In 1980, the delta antigen was recognized as a component of a pathogen whose replication depended on an obligatory

R. Fawaz (✉)
Children's Hospital Boston, 300 Longwood Avenue, Boston, MA 02115, USA
e-mail: Rima.Fawaz@childrens.harvard.edu

M.M. Jonas (ed.), *Viral Hepatitis in Children: Unique Features and Opportunities*, Clinical Gastroenterology, DOI 10.1007/978-1-60761-373-2_6,

coinfection with hepatitis B virus (HBV) [2, 3]. In 1986, hepatitis D virus (HDV) was cloned and sequenced [4–6].

Description

Hepatitis D virus is the only member of the Deltaviridae family [7]. It is a 36-nm spherical particle composed of an RNA genome, a single HDV antigen, and a lipoprotein envelope from Hepatitis B virus (HBV). The HDV genome is a single-stranded RNA 1672–1697 nucleotides in size [8]. It is the only known animal virus with a circular RNA genome [7]. It shares structural properties with plant viruses, such as viroids and virusoids [9]. Due to a high degree of intramolecular complementarity, the genome collapses to form an unbranched, double-stranded, stable rod-like structure [10]. The HDV genome encodes its single and only nucleocapsid protein, the HDV antigen. Based on genomic heterogeneity, a classification into eight major genotypes has been proposed [8, 11, 12]. Genotype 1 is the most ubiquitous and is present throughout the world. Genotype 2 is more commonly found in Japan and Taiwan and genotype 3 has been associated with outbreaks in Venezuela and Peru [13].

The hepatitis D antigen (HDAg) is present within the internal nucleocapsid. Approximately 70 copies of HDAg in its two forms, short form (S-HDAg) and long form (L-HDAg), are complexed to the HDV RNA to form a ribonucleoprotein structure [14]. The two forms are identical except for a 19 amino acid C-terminus. The S-HDAg is 195 amino acids in length and is required for HDV RNA replication. The L-HDAg is 214 amino acids in length; it suppresses RNA replication and is required for virion assembly [7, 14]. The outer envelope of HDV is provided by hepatitis B virus (HBV) and is composed of lipids and all three forms of hepatitis B surface antigen (HBsAg). The proportion of different forms of HBsAg in the envelope of HDV is different from that of the hepatitis B virion [7]. HDV can replicate autonomously, but to produce infection and clinical illnesses the presence of active HBV infection is obligatory [15, 16].

Epidemiology

Seroprevalence studies of anti-HD in HBV carriers reveal a worldwide but a non-uniform distribution that does not parallel that of HBV. It is estimated that around 5% of HBV carriers may be co-infected with HDV, bringing the prevalence to about 15 million people worldwide [17]. However, as with other hepatitis viruses, the incidence is decreasing due to improvement in hygiene, economic standards, increased awareness of transmission of infectious diseases, and, very importantly, universal vaccination for hepatitis B [18–20]. In Italy, where hepatitis D was first described, the prevalence of HDV has decreased from 23% in 1987 to 14% in 1992 to 8.3% in 1997 [20, 21]. Similar declines in prevalence have also been reported in Spain, Turkey, and Taiwan [22–24].

More recent reports from Europe indicate that the prevalence of HDV in the last 10 years has not continued to decline and there are still pockets of high prevalence.

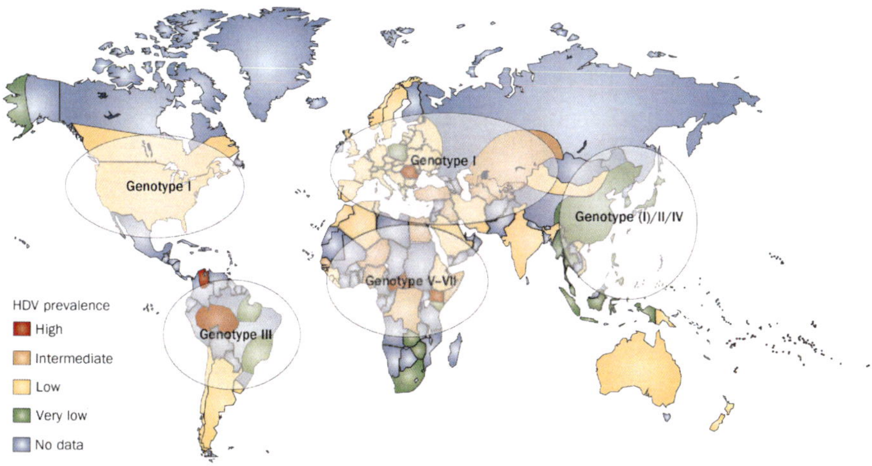

Fig. 1 Global epidemiology of HDV infection according to viral genotype. HDV genotype 1 is the most frequent genotype and is distributed throughout the world, especially in Europe, the Middle East, North America, and North Africa. By contrast, HDV genotype 2 is observed in the Far East, and HDV genotype 3 is seen exclusively in the northern part of South America. Abbreviation: *HDV* hepatitis D virus. (From: Wedemeyer and Manns. *Nat Rev Gastroenterol Hepatol.* Jan;7(1):31–40. Printed with permission from Nature reviews)

This is mainly due to two populations: those that are chronically infected and are ageing, and those that migrate from high endemic areas of the world and contribute to local spread of the infection [25–27]. There continue to be pockets of high prevalence of hepatitis D in the Middle East, central Africa, and northern parts of South America [8] (Fig. 1).

Epidemiological patterns worldwide depend on the route of transmission. In the Mediterranean basin, infection is most commonly transmitted by close personal contact and tends to occur early in life [21, 28]. In Europe and North America, infection is most commonly transmitted by exposure to blood and blood products, so high-risk groups include intravenous drug users and multiply transfused patients [26]. In the Far East, infection tends to occur either by sexual transmission or with intravenous drug use [13]. Vertical transmission and transmission of HDV in homosexual men who are HBsAg positive are rare [29].

Epidemiology of HDV infection in children parallels that in adults. Intrafamilial spread plays an important role in endemic areas as demonstrated by almost identical HDV strains in members from the same family [30, 31].

Clinical Features

HDV infection can only occur in the presence of HBV infection, either as coinfection or as superinfection. Coinfection occurs when acquisition of HBV and HDV are simultaneous. The clinical picture simulates that of classical acute HBV infection.

Depending on the HBV titer, the incubation period is typically 3–7 weeks. The pre-icteric phase usually lasts 3–7 days, during which fever, anorexia, nausea, fatigue, and malaise predominate. This is accompanied by elevated aminotransferases. The icteric phase that follows is manifested by jaundice, hepatosplenomegaly, pruritus, dark urine, and clay colored stools. These signs may persist for 1–2 months. During the convalescent phase, symptoms resolve. Coinfection with HBV and HDV is usually transient and self-limited, although severe fulminant hepatic failure can occur. Progression to chronic infection parallels that after acute hepatitis B infection alone and occurs in less than 10% of coinfected individuals [13, 32] (Fig. 2).

Superinfection occurs when individuals with established chronic HBV are superinfected with HDV. This can present as severe icteric hepatitis in an undiagnosed HBV carrier or as an exacerbation of stable chronic hepatitis B. In the acute picture, it may rapidly lead to fulminant hepatic failure at a frequency ten times higher than that of other forms of viral hepatitis [33]. Superinfection leads to chronic HDV in 75–97% of cases [34, 35]. This usually has three phases: acute, chronic, and late phases. The acute phase is characterized by high alanine aminotransferase (ALT) levels, active HDV replication, and suppression of HBsAg and HBV DNA. During the chronic phase, ALT levels decrease but may remain moderately elevated, HDV replication decreases, and HBV reactivation at low levels may occur. The late phase is characterized by reduced levels of both viruses and development of cirrhosis [35] (Fig. 2).

The natural history of chronic HDV infection is that of an asymptomatic carrier state in approximately 15% of cases and severe progressive disease in up to 85% of individuals [36]. Although cirrhosis may remain stable for many years, the risk of morbidity and mortality with chronic HBV and HDV is much higher than that with HBV cirrhosis alone [37]. Progression to cirrhosis with chronic HDV typically takes 5–10 years but can occur as early as 2 years after infection [33]. A recent observational study from Milan tracked the course of 299 HDV infected individuals for up to 28 years (mean 20 years). Patients with persistent HDV replication developed cirrhosis at a 4% annual rate and hepatocellular carcinoma (HCC) at 2.8% per year. Of the patients with cirrhosis, 25% developed HCC during follow-up. Liver failure was the cause of death in 59% of the patients [38]. A similar study from Taiwan revealed that survival of patients with genotype 1 HDV was 50% after 15 years. They also found that dual infection with HBV and HDV, older age, genotype 1 HDV, and genotype C HBV correlated with adverse outcomes [39]. Factors proven to influence the course of the HDV-related liver disease are HDV genotype and coinfection with other viruses such as HIV and HCV [40, 41].

Fig. 2 (continued) (**b**) Serological events during hepatitis B virus (HBV) and hepatitis D virus (HDV) superinfection. If an individual already infected with HBV is infected with HDV, there is a marked elevation of alanine transaminase (ALT) coincident with the onset of symptoms and the onset of jaundice. HDV RNA also can be detected at the onset of symptoms. ALT levels fluctuate over the next few months as IgM anti-HDV decreases and total anti-HDV rises. Throughout the course of HDV superinfection, hepatitis B surface antigen (HBsAg) remains detectable. (From: Feigin and Cherry's Textbook of Pediatric Infectious Diseases, 6th edition, 2009. Printed with permission from Elsevier Health)

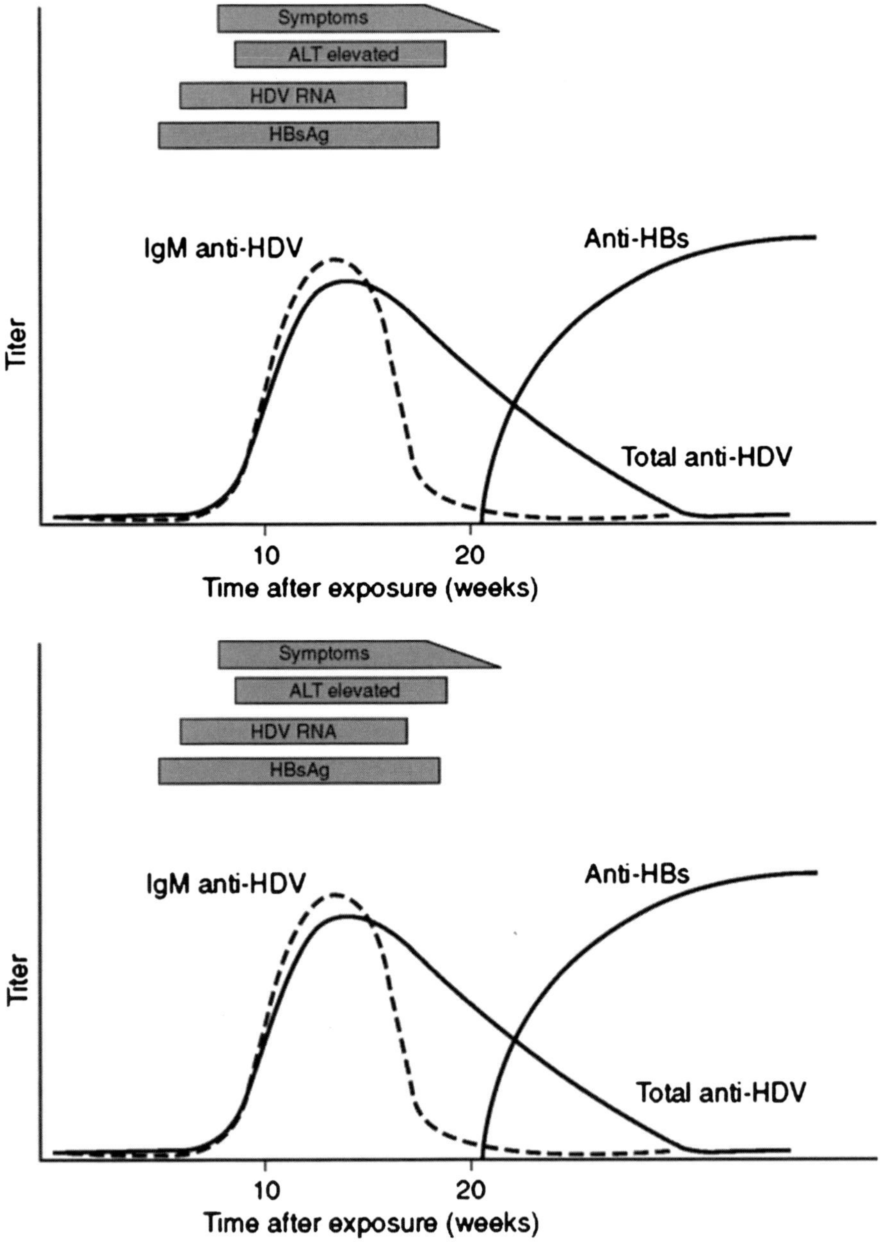

Fig. 2 (**a**) Serological events during hepatitis B virus (HBV) and hepatitis D virus (HDV) coinfection that resolves. After exposure to both viruses, hepatitis B surface antigen (HBsAg) and HDV RNA can be detected shortly before the onset of symptoms. Serum alanine transaminase (ALT) is elevated for the duration of detectable serum HDV RNA and HBsAg. Serum IgM anti-HDV rises when symptoms are present and falls as HDV infection resolves, and the anti-HBs titer becomes elevated. When both infections have resolved, anti-HBs is detectable in serum, but total anti-HDV is very low. (From: Feigin and Cherry's Textbook of Pediatric Infectious Diseases, 6th edition, 2009. Printed with permission from Elsevier Health).

Genotype 1 is the predominant HDV genotype worldwide and seems to be associated with a higher incidence of acute liver failure following acute hepatitis D, a lower remission rate and increased incidence of adverse outcomes compared to genotype 2 [35, 39, 42]. Genotype 3 has been associated with outbreaks of acute hepatitis D with a high incidence of fulminant hepatic failure in South America [43–45]. While the HDV genotype may influence the efficiency of the assembly of HBsAg into the HDV virion, the HBV genotype seems to be less important for this process [46].

Hepatitis D in Children

Superimposed delta infection profoundly modifies the natural history of chronic hepatitis B in children and converts a usually mild disease into a severe hepatitis with a propensity to progression [47]. Severe cases of hepatitis in children reported from different parts of the world were discovered to be caused by HDV superinfection. In these series, there was a higher incidence of fulminant hepatic failure in young children [44, 48]. The incidence of hepatitis D in children has decreased with the implementation of the universal hepatitis B vaccination programs, as evident in adults. However, there continue to be outbreaks reported in children in hepatitis B hyper-endemic areas of the world [49] as well as pockets of high seroprevalence reaching up to 9% [50]. Vertical transmission is rare because HBV/HDV-infected mothers are usually anti-HBe positive and thus have lower levels of HBV viremia. Perinatal transmission does occur in circumstances that permit HBV transmission such as high maternal HBe antigenemia and high HBV DNA viremia [51].

Pathogenesis

The mechanisms of liver injury in HDV infection are not fully understood. Clinical evidence points to an immune-mediated disease process, especially in chronic infection, whereas direct cytopathic damage has been implicated during acute infection [52, 53].

Liver histology is usually similar to that of hepatitis B. Histological activity in the liver seems to be weakly correlated with serum levels of HBsAg and not with HDV viremia [54]. In fact, some investigators have found a negative correlation between HDV viremia and fibrosis scores, supporting the concept that immune response and not cytopathic effect plays the major role in liver injury [55].

Diagnosis

The presence of HBsAg is necessary for the diagnosis of HDV infection. Testing for HDV should be carried out in any patient with severe unexplained hepatitis or in a patient with known risk factors that predispose to acquiring infectious hepatitis,

Table 1 Hepatitis D virus infection: diagnostic patterns

	Acute HDV/HBV coinfection	Acute HDV superinfection	Chronic HDV infection
HBsAg	+	+	+
Anti-HBc IgM	+	–	–
Serum HDAg	+/–	+/–	–
Anti-HDV IgM	+	++	+++
Anti-HDV IgG	+/–	++	+++
HDV RNA	+	+	+++
Liver HDAg	+	+	+/–

HDV hepatitis D virus, *HBV* hepatitis B virus, *HBsAg* hepatitis B surface antigen, *IgM* immunoglobulin M, *HDAg* hepatitis D antigen, *IgG* immunoglobulin G

such as history of intravenous drug abuse, promiscuous sexual practices, exposure to blood or blood products, household members with known HBV or HDV.

Serum HDAg can be detected by microplate-based, enzyme-linked (EIA) or radioimmunoassay (RIA). These assays are not commercially available in the USA. Early testing for serum HDAg in the acute setting may yield negative results and repeat testing may be necessary [56–58]. In the chronic setting, HDAg levels are usually low as they are complexed with anti-HDV that is circulating in high titers (Table 1).

Anti-HDV antibodies develop in every individual infected with HDV [59]. Therefore, direct testing for HDV RNA in the absence of anti-HDV antibodies is probably not useful. However, the presence of anti-HDV antibodies does not necessarily indicate active infection, as the antibodies may persist for years after recovery from infection [60]. HDV infection should be confirmed by testing for HDV RNA.

Assays for anti-HDV antibodies are EIAs or RIAs. Total anti-HDV antibody is the only commercially available test for use in clinical practice in the USA. The antibody typically appears about 4 weeks after acute infection [56, 61]. In acute self-limited HDV infection, the initial antibody is anti-HDV IgM, which appears at 4 weeks and is usually transient. Anti-HDV IgM may appear briskly and last for longer duration in chronic HDV infection. In this setting, the antibody may correlate with HDV replication and disease severity [56, 62]. Anti-HDV IgG is present in high titers in chronic infection and correlates well with ongoing HDV replication, so the presence of this antibody does not indicate resolved infection, and the antibody does not confer protection. In resolved HDV, anti-HDV is usually present in low titers. HBV/ HDV coinfection may be discriminated from HDV superinfection of chronic HBV by the detection of IgM hepatitis B core antibody (Table 1).

Testing for HDV RNA in serum is carried out by either molecular hybridization or by reverse transcriptase-polymerase chain reaction (RT-PCR)-based assays. RT-PCR assays have a lower limit of detection of 10 genomes per ml [63–65]. HDV RNA is an early and sensitive marker of acute HDV and is useful to follow and assess resolution of HDV infection. This test should be used to confirm active infection in individuals seropositive for anti-HDV.

Finally, HDV can be diagnosed by detection of HDAg or HDV RNA in liver tissue. HDAg detection in liver tissue is performed by direct immunofluorescence or immunohistochemical staining. The presence of HDAg was considered the gold standard to diagnose ongoing infection, but in patients with cirrhosis, the levels may be too low to detect [35]. Liver biopsies continue to be strongly advocated by some authors as a key component of the diagnostic workup [59].

HDV genotyping is performed by some research laboratories and may help to identify patients at increased risk of developing end-stage liver disease [39]. However, its use in the routine clinical setting is not recommended.

The distinction between HBV/HDV coinfection and HDV superinfection depends on the presence of hepatitis B core (HBc) IgM in the former. When there is clinically acute hepatitis, the typical findings include a positive HDAg, anti-HDV IgM antibodies, and HDV RNA. The diagnosis of chronic hepatitis D is made by positive HBsAg and elevated ALT for more than 6 months, anti-HDV antibodies or HDV RNA, and if possible a liver biopsy with HDAg positivity in hepatocytes and a concomitant necroinflammatory disease (Fig. 2). Patients with chronic HDV may develop antibodies of the IgA subtype to HDV [34, 66]. In a small study, IgA anti-HDV correlated independently with moderate-to-severe histological activity. The role of this antibody in liver damage is unknown [66].

In children with acute hepatitis, there is no need to routinely assess for HDV infection. Testing may be considered in children with unusually severe and protracted hepatitis documented to be positive to HBV, in those with an acute exacerbation of stable chronic HBV, in those with known family history of HDV, and in children who emigrated from countries with high prevalence of HDV.

Treatment

There is no established treatment for chronic hepatitis D. The natural history of this disease and the uniqueness of the delta virus make it a difficult target for therapy. Although interferon alpha (INF-α) was first used in the treatment of chronic HDV 25 years ago, it remains the only approved therapy for HDV today [67].

Both pilot and randomized studies have shown that therapy with IFN-α can ameliorate chronic hepatitis D. The mechanism of action of IFN in HDV treatment is unclear, but is thought to be due to either its inhibitory effects on HBV or its immunomodulatory effects, as it does not exhibit any antiviral activity against HDV in vitro [68, 69]. Its efficacy is related to both the dose and the duration of therapy. Standard doses have clearly been shown to be inferior to high doses of IFN-α. In a small randomized control trial in adults of 3 million units versus 9 million units of IFN-α three times a week for 48 weeks, normal ALT levels were achieved in 29% and undetectable HDV RNA in 21% of those who received standard dosing, compared to 71% normal ALT and 50% undetectable HDV RNA in individuals who received the higher dose. In addition, treatment with the high dose was associated with improved histological outcome and benefit in long-term survival even after 10 years. Unfortunately, almost all patients relapsed with positive HDV RNA after stopping treatment [70, 71]. It seems that 2 years of therapy is superior to shorter duration of therapy for HDV RNA clearance [72], but this is not a consistent finding [73]. Pegylated interferon (PEG-IFN) appears to be more effective than standard interferon in the treatment of chronic HDV, as shown in three small trials published in 2006. In one study, the use of PEG-IFN-α_{2b} at 1.5 mcg/kg weekly for 12 months resulted in a 43% (6 of 14) sustained viral response (SVR) defined as undetectable serum HDV RNA 6 months after therapy [74]. However, in a similar study in which 12 patients were treated with the same protocol, SVR was obtained in only 17% [75]. In the third study, 38 patients received PEG-IFN-α_{2b} for 72 weeks and 22 of those also received ribavirin for the first 48 weeks; SVR was achieved in only 21% [76]. Notably, ribavirin had no beneficial effect on SVR. In the Hep-Net International Delta Hepatitis Interventional Trial (HIDIT-1) that included 90 patients randomized to receive 180 mcg of PEG-IFN-α_{2a} weekly plus either 10 mg of adefovir dipivoxil or placebo daily or 10 mg of adefovir dipivoxil alone for 48 weeks, SVR was obtained in 25% of patients in the PEG-IFN arms but none in the adefovir monotherapy arm. Importantly, combination therapy of PEG-IFN with adefovir had no advantages in the reduction of serum HBV DNA or HDV RNA levels [77].

Treatments using different nucleoside and nucleotide analogs, such as lamivudine [78–80] and ribavirin [76, 81, 82] therapy have yielded disappointing results.

Treatment in children has been just as unsatisfactory as in adults. A small German study of eight children treated with IFN-α revealed improvement in serum aminotransferases and an earlier seroconversion to anti-HBe compared to historical controls, but no effect on HDV parameters [83]. A similar Greek study of seven children treated with IFN-α, 3 million units three times a week for 1 year, revealed a decrease in serum aminotransferases but no improvement in liver histology. All children remained anti-HDV positive and four children had persistent HDV RNA at the end of the treatment [84]. At this time, there are no established recommendations regarding treatment for children with chronic HDV.

Prevention

The only effective measures to control the spread of HDV infection are counseling against high-risk behaviors among individuals with chronic hepatitis B infection and universal vaccination with hepatitis B vaccine for all other individuals. Passive immunoprophylaxis with hepatitis B immunoglobulin does not confer any protection against HDV infection, unless it controls the spread of HBV infection [85]. Therefore, the use of HBIG in the post-exposure setting in a known chronic hepatitis B carrier is ineffective. In children, universal vaccination remains the cornerstone of prevention. It is prudent to check adequate immunity to HBV after vaccination in children with household members known to have HDV infection to inhibit intrafamilial transmission.

Hepatitis E

Hepatitis E was previously referred to as enterically transmitted non-A and non-B (NANB) hepatitis. It was first identified as distinct human disease in 1983 when virus-like particles were identified by immune electron microscopy in the stools of a volunteer orally infected with pooled stool extracts from presumed cases of epidemic NANB hepatitis. The disease was subsequently transmitted in an experimental animal model [86]. In 1988, the causative agent of NANB was named hepatitis E. The genome of this virus was cloned in 1990 and fully sequenced in 1991 [87–89].

Description

Hepatitis E virus (HEV) is a nonenveloped, icosahedral particle, 27–34 nm in diameter. It contains a single-stranded, positive sense RNA genome approximately 7.5 kb in length [86, 90, 91]. It was considered a member of the Calciviridae family from 1988 to 1998 [92, 93], but was reclassified into a class of its own of the genus Hepevirus in the family Hepeviridae. The viral genome consists of short non-coding regions at both the 5′ and 3′ ends, and three large open reading frames (ORF). ORF1 is the largest, consisting of 1693 codons, and encodes for nonstructural proteins responsible for replication of the viral genome and processing of the viral polyprotein. ORF2 consists of 660 codons and codes for structural proteins. ORF3 is composed of 123 codons and codes for a small cytoskeleton-associated phosphoprotein with uncertain function [89]. ORF2 overlaps ORF3 but neither overlap ORF1.

Based on phylogenetic analysis, a classification into four genotypes and 24 subtypes has been proposed [94]. Genotypes 1 and 2 appear to infect only humans, while genotypes 3 and 4 infect both humans and animals. The correlation of genotype to clinical features is not well understood.

Each genotype appears to have a geographical distribution. Genotype 1 has been isolated from epidemic and sporadic cases in Asia and Africa. Isolates from these regions have 90% or more nucleotide sequence homology [94]. Genotype 2 has been isolated from outbreaks in Mexico and western Africa. These isolates have nucleotide homology of 75% with genotype 1 [94–96]. Genotype 3 has been associated with less virulent disease and has been reported in the USA, as well as in several industrialized countries such as Europe, Japan, Australia, New Zealand, Korea, and Argentina. Isolates from these regions have also 74–75% nucleotide homology to isolates from genotypes 1 and 2 [94, 97]. Genotype 4 has been reported in sporadic cases from China, Taiwan, Japan, and Vietnam [94, 98] (Fig. 3).

Epidemiology

The epidemiology of hepatitis E is similar to that of hepatitis A as its predominant route of transmission is fecal-oral, but hepatitis A is more easily transmitted and has

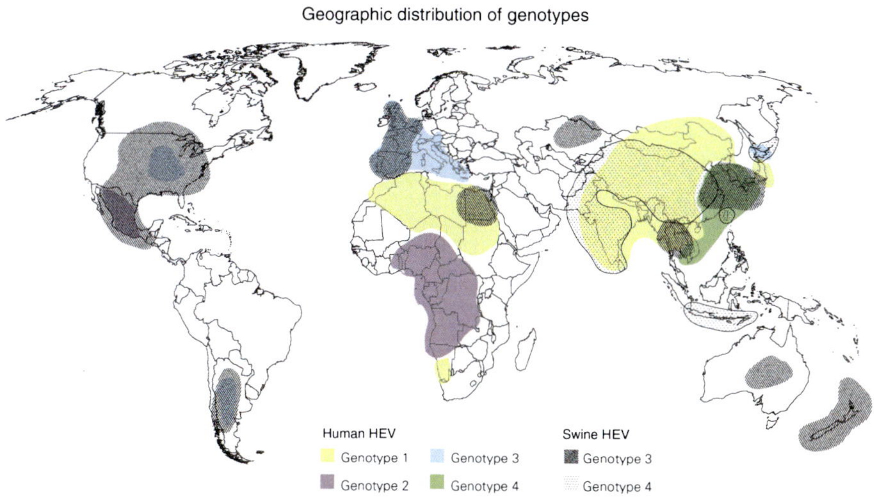

Fig. 3 Map showing geographic distribution of hepatitis E virus genotypes among (**a**) human isolates, and (**b**) swine isolates. (From Aggarwal and Naik S. *J Gastroenterol Hepatol.* Sep 2009;24(9):1484–1493. Printed with permission from John Wiley and Sons)

a wider worldwide distribution. The highest incidence of hepatitis E infection is found in areas of lower standards of sanitation that promote transmission of the virus. Transmission most commonly occurs by fecally contaminated water or through contaminated food. HEV has the highest attack rate in the age groups 15–40 years, with overall attack rates ranging from 3 to 30% in adults and 0.2–10% in children [99–102]. This is possibly due to the fact that most children have anicteric and asymptomatic disease. In one report, seroprevalence data were the same across all childhood groups (0–5, 6–11, and 11–18 years) and was not different from those of adults. This might imply that infection during childhood may not confer lasting immunity [103]. HEV is less commonly transmitted person to person, with secondary attack rates reported as low as 0.7–2.2% [104, 105]. Transmission has been reported to occur by blood transfusions in endemic areas [106–108] and by the maternal-fetal route [109].

HEV continues to be epidemic in Asia, Africa, Middle East, and Central America [110–113]. There have been an increasing number of autochthonous (locally acquired) cases in recent years in developed countries. Until recently, sporadic HEV infections were generally rare and mainly related to travel, but more recently non-travel cases caused by zoonotic genotypes 3 and 4 have been reported [114]. Risk factors for sporadic cases include consumption of shellfish or animal meats and direct contact with infected animals [114–117]. This is supported by the high seroprevalence of anti-HEV antibodies among individuals with occupational contact with swine [118–120]. This was also highlighted by the results from the Third National Health and Nutrition Examination Survey evaluating 18,695 sera obtained during the period from 1988 to 1994. There was a surprisingly high seroprevalence rate of 21% for anti-HEV IgG antibodies in the civilian non-institutionalized US population. It was concluded that having pets and consuming organ meats may play a role in acquisition of HEV. Other hypotheses to explain the discrepancy between clinically apparent hepatitis E and seroprevalence estimates include the possibility of anicteric disease caused by the less-virulent genotype 3, underreporting, or nonspecificity of the assays used [121].

Vertical Transmission

There are limited data regarding vertical transmission of HEV but when it does occur, it seems to be associated with significant morbidity and mortality in the infants. In one report, six out of eight babies born to mothers infected with hepatitis E in their third trimester had clinical and serologic evidence of HEV infection soon after birth. Two of the eight babies were born with hypoglycemia and hypothermia, and died within 24 h; one had massive hepatic necrosis [122]. In another report, all 26 babies born to mothers HEV-RNA positive at the time of delivery developed acute HEV-RNA associated hepatitis. Two of the 26 babies had early onset of hypoglycemia and hypothermia and died within 48 h of birth [123].

Clinical Features

The clinical manifestations of HEV infection are similar to those of other types of viral hepatitis, although the disease seems to more severe when compared to hepatitis A infection [124]. It is usually a self-limited acute disease but HEV can cause acute liver failure (ALF), especially in pregnant women [125] and those with preexisting liver disease [126, 127]. Acute HEV infection does not develop into chronic hepatitis E except in a few select settings in immunocompromised hosts [128–130].

Typically HEV infection manifests as acute icteric hepatitis in adolescents and adults. The incubation period ranges from 2 to 10 weeks but usually is around 40 days. The prodromal phase, lasting 1–4 days, is associated with flu-like symptoms, fever, mild chills, abdominal pain, anorexia, nausea, vomiting, diarrhea, arthralgias, and a transient macular rash. These symptoms are followed by jaundice, dark urine, clay-colored stools, and sometimes pruritus. The prodromal symptoms usually subside, except for the gastrointestinal symptoms which may persist for a longer time [100, 111, 131]. Prolonged cholestasis can occur in up to 60% of patients [124]. Physical examination usually reveals jaundice with mild hepatomegaly and 25% of patients will have soft splenomegaly. Laboratory evaluation reveals marked elevation of aminotransferases and gamma glutamyltransferase activity with modest elevation of alkaline phosphatase and a variable increase in conjugated bilirubin. The elevation of the aminotransferases may precede the symptoms and reaches a peak by the end of the first week. The liver tests return to normal by 6 weeks [131, 132] (Fig. 4).

In children, HEV infection is usually asymptomatic or anicteric [133, 134]. HEV infection in pregnant women has classically been thought to have a higher

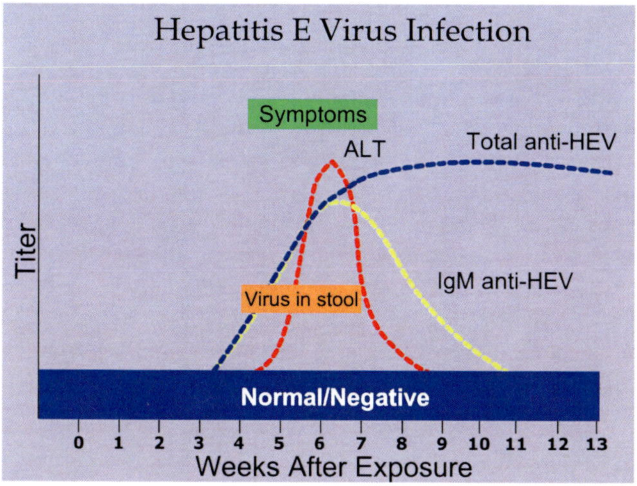

Fig. 4 Hepatitis E. Reproduced from: Centers for Disease Control and Prevention: http://www.cdc.gov/hepatitis/Resources/Professionals/Training/Serology/training.htm#one

morbidity and mortality, especially in the third trimester, with a case fatality rate reaching 15–25% compared to 0.2–4% in the general population [92, 125]. Reasons for this are unknown, but one possible explanation is that pregnancy appears to increase viral replication [135]. Supporting data show that pregnant women with acute icteric HEV hepatitis have a higher mortality rate and worse obstetric and fetal outcome compared to pregnant women with acute icteric hepatitis by other viruses [136]. One retrospective study demonstrated that the outcome of HEV-related ALF was independent of sex, pregnancy, or trimester status, and mortality ranged from 53 to 59%; in other words, once ALF is established, the outcome is the same in the pregnant patient as compared to an age-matched population [137].

The general rule for HEV infection is self-resolution without progression to chronicity. However, in 2008, three publications demonstrated that chronic infection with HEV can be established in the immunocompromised setting. In one study, fourteen cases of acute HEV were identified after solid organ transplant. Eight patients developed chronic hepatitis E confirmed by persistently elevated aminotransferases, persistent HEV RNA in serum, and histological features of chronic hepatitis [129]. Another paper documented two cases of chronic HEV after liver transplantation, both with genotype 3, that progressed to cirrhosis and ultimately required retransplantation, [128]. The third paper reported two cases of rapidly progressive HEV-associated cirrhosis in kidney transplant patients [138]. In 2009, two separate case reports described chronic HEV infection; one in a patient with non-Hodgkin lymphoma receiving rituximab [130] and another in a patient with human immunodeficiency virus infection [139].

Pathogenesis

The mechanisms of liver injury in hepatitis E are unknown but are thought to be due to an immune-mediated process, as infiltrating lymphocytes are of the cytotoxic/suppressor immunophenotype, and hepatocyte cultures inoculated with HEV do not show any cytopathic change [140]. Liver histology is slightly different from other types of viral hepatitis as more than half the cases have cholestatic hepatitis. In these patients, canalicular bile stasis and gland-like transformation of the hepatocytes predominate and degenerative changes of the parenchymal cells are less evident [141, 142]. In some cases, changes are similar to those seen with other types of viral hepatitis, such as ballooning and acidophilic degeneration of hepatocytes and confluent hepatic necrosis [141]. Histopathological findings in the liver in children with HEV infection are similar to those in adults.

Diagnosis

The diagnosis of HEV infection depends on detection of virus-specific immune response in the host or detection of the virus in the blood or stool by PCR. There are no commercially available assays for clinical practice in the USA to diagnose HEV infection. However, testing can be performed by research laboratories through the Centers for Disease Control and Prevention.

Testing for anti-HEV infection was historically done by immune electron microscopy and fluorescent antibody-blocking assays. Currently, Western blot assays and enzyme immunoassays (EIAs) are used for detection of IgM and IgG antibodies against HEV. IgM anti-HEV appears in the early phase of the illness and is positive in 90% of sera collected within 1 week to 2 months after the onset of symptoms [143–145]. Assays to detect IgM anti-HEV are usually reliable when used during acute hepatitis in endemic areas but have not been validated in the diagnosis of acute HEV infection in low-incidence areas. IgG anti-HEV persists for years after acquisition of HEV infection, but the true duration is unknown [145]. Both the above assays used for diagnosis of IgG anti-HEV have variable sensitivity rates; hence the use of nucleic acid testing by PCR is the gold standard [146].

Treatment

There is currently no specific antiviral therapy for HEV infection. Passive immunoprophylaxis has shown benefit in laboratory animals inoculated with HEV, but not in human studies using either pre- or post-exposure immunoglobulins [147–149]. Treatment as in other forms of viral hepatitis consists of supportive therapy, mainly restriction of activity, ensuring adequate hydration and nutrition, and avoidance of any hepatotoxic medications.

Prevention

Prevention of hepatitis E depends on good sanitation and the availability of clean drinking water. During epidemics, efforts to improve water quality have led to a decline in the number of new cases [150, 151]. Isolation of infected individuals is usually not indicated as person-to-person transmission is very low [152]; however, shedding of the virus in the stool can continue up to 14 days after the onset of jaundice [86, 153].

HEV Vaccines

In animal studies, the use of HEV capsid proteins and HEV DNA has resulted in the induction of virus-specific protective antibodies [154–157]. Human vaccines are not commercially available yet. In a large placebo-controlled trial of one vaccine developed using a 56-kD truncated HEV ORF2, the efficacy rate was 95% after completion of three doses and 86% after two doses [158]. The study, however, had the limitation of including only healthy young male volunteers (Nepalese Army soldiers), so more studies would be needed to evaluate safety and efficacy in pregnant women, children, and those with pre-existing liver disease. In addition, the primary outcome was the clinical disease rate and not the infection rate. Lastly, anti-HEV titers at the end of the study decreased to below protective levels in 44% of individuals, and hence further assessment of long-term protection is needed [156, 158]. A phase II trial of a different vaccine preparation using a truncated HEV capsid protein has been reported [159].

The role of HEV vaccines in prevention of disease remains unclear. This will ultimately depend on the duration of protection offered by the vaccine, the ability of the vaccine to prevent transmission of disease, and the cost of the vaccine [160]. For now, prevention remains key, and encouraging good hygiene practices should be emphasized. For travelers to endemic areas, basic food hygiene precautions should be exercised. These include avoidance of drinking water or ice of unknown sources as well as uncooked food, fruits, or vegetables.

References

1. Rizzetto M, Canese MG, Arico S, et al. Immunofluorescence detection of new antigen-antibody system (delta/anti-delta) associated to hepatitis B virus in liver and in serum of HBsAg carriers. Gut 1977;18(12):997–1003.
2. Rizzetto M, Canese MG, Gerin JL, London WT, Sly DL, Purcell RH. Transmission of the hepatitis B virus-associated delta antigen to chimpanzees. J Infect Dis. 1980;141(5): 590–602.
3. Rizzetto M, Hoyer B, Canese MG, Shih JW, Purcell RH, Gerin JL. delta Agent: association of delta antigen with hepatitis B surface antigen and RNA in serum of delta-infected chimpanzees. Proc Natl Acad Sci U S A. 1980;77(10):6124–6128.

4. Wang KS, Choo QL, Weiner AJ, et al. Structure, sequence and expression of the hepatitis delta (delta) viral genome. Nature. 1986;323(6088):508–514.
5. Kos A, Dijkema R, Arnberg AC, van der Meide PH, Schellekens H. The hepatitis delta (delta) virus possesses a circular RNA. Nature. 1986;323(6088):558–560.
6. Chen PJ, Kalpana G, Goldberg J, et al. Structure and replication of the genome of the hepatitis delta virus. Proc Natl Acad Sci U S A. 1986;83(22):8774–8778.
7. Lai MM. The molecular biology of hepatitis delta virus. Annu Rev Biochem. 1995;64:259–286.
8. Radjef N, Gordien E, Ivaniushina V, Gault E, Anais P, Drugan T, et al. Molecular phylogenetic analyses indicate a wide and ancient rediation of African hepatitis delta virus, suggesting a deltavirus genus of at least seven major clades. J Virol. 2004;78:2537–2544.
9. Branch AD, Robertson HD. A replication cycle for viroids and other small infectious RNA's. Science. 1984;223(4635):450–455.
10. Taylor J NF, Rizetto M. Hepatitis delta virus: from structure to disease expression. Rev Med Virol. 1992;2:161–167.
11. Le Gal F Gault E, Ripault MP, Serpaggi J, Trinchet JC, Gordien E, Deny P. Eighth major clade for hepatitis delta virus. Emerg Infect Dis. 2006;12(9):1447–1450.
12. Deny P. Hepatitis delta virus genetic variability: from genotypes I, II, III to eight major clades? Curr Top Microbiol Immunol. 2006;307:151–171.
13. Hadziyannis S. Review: hepatitis delta. J Gastroenterol and Hepatol. 1997;12(4):289–298.
14. Ryu WS, Netter H, Bayer M et al. Ribonucleoprotein complexes of hepatitis delta virus. J Virol. 1993;67(6):3281–8287.
15. Binchko V, Netter HJ, Wu TT, et. a. Pathogenesis associated with replication of hepatitis delta virus. Infect Agents Dis. 1994;3(2–3):94–97.
16. Jacobsen IM, Dienstag J. The delta hepatitis agent: viral hepatitis, type D. Gastroenterology. 1984;86:1614–1616.
17. Rizzetto M, Durazzo M. Hepatitis Delta virus(HDV) infections. Epidemiological and clinical heterogeneity. J Hepatol. 1991;13(Suppl 4):S116–S118.
18. Rosina F, Conoscitore P, Cuppone R, et al. Changing pattern of chronic hepatitis D in southern Europe. Gastroenterology. 1999;117:161–166.
19. Navascues C, Rodriguez M, Sottorio N, et al. Epidemiology of hepatitis D virus infection: changes in the last 14 years. Am J Gastroenterol. 1995;90:1981–1984.
20. Gaeta GB, Stroffolini T, Chiaramonte M, et al. Chronic hepatitis D: a vanishing disease? An italian multicenter study. Hepatology. 2000;32:824–827.
21. Sagnelli E, Stroffolini T, Ascione A, et al. Decrease in HDV endemicity in Italy. J Hepatol. 1997;26(1):20–24.
22. Navascues CA, Rodriguez M, Sotorrio NG, et al. Epidemiology of hepatitis D virus infection: changes in the last 14 years. Am J Gastroenterol. 1995;90(11):1981–1984.
23. Degertekin H, Yalcin K, Yakut M. The prevalence of hepatitis delta virus infection in acute and chronic liver diseases in Turkey: an analysis of clinical studies. Turk J Gastroenterol. 2006;17(1): 25–34.
24. Huo TI, Wu JC, Lin RY, Sheng WY, Chang FY, Lee SD. Decreasing hepatitis D virus infection in Taiwan: an analysis of contributory factors. J Gastroenterol Hepatol. 1997;12(11):747–751.
25. Cross TJ, Rizzi P, Horner M, et al. The increasing prevalence of hepatitis delta virus (HDV) infection in South London. J Med Virol. 2008;80(2):277–282.
26. Wedemeyer H, Heidrich B, Manns MP. Hepatitis D virus infection – not a vanishing disease in Europe! Hepatology. 2007;45(5):1331–1332.
27. Gaeta GB, Stroffolini T, Smedile A, Niro G, Mele A. Hepatitis delta in Europe: vanishing or refreshing? Hepatology. 2007;46(4):1312–1313.
28. Stroffolini T, Ferrigno L, Cialdea L, et al. Incidence and risk factors of acute Delta hepatitis in Italy: results from a national surveillance system. SEIEVA Collaborating Group. J Hepatol. 1994;21(6):1123–1126.
29. Weisfuse IB, Hadler SC, Fields HA, et al. Delta hepatitis in homosexual men in the United States. Hepatology. 1989;9(6):872–874.

30. Niro GA, Casey JL, Gravinese E, et al. Intrafamilial transmission of hepatitis delta virus: molecular evidence. J Hepatol. 1999;30(4):564–569.
31. Hsu HY, Chang MH, Chen DS, Lee CY. Hepatitis D virus infection in children with acute or chronic hepatitis B virus infection in Taiwan. J Pediatr. 1988;112(6):888–892.
32. Smedile A, Farci P, Verme G, et al. Influence of delta infection on severity of hepatitis B. Lancet. 1982;2(8305):945–947.
33. Percell RH, Gerin JL. Hepatitis Delta Virus. In: Fields BN, Knipe DM, Howley PM, ed. Fields Virology. 3rd ed. Philadelphia: Lippincott-Raven; 1996:2819–2829.
34. Hoofnagle JH. Type D (delta) hepatitis. JAMA. 1989;261(9):1321–1325.
35. Wu JC, Chen TZ, Huang YS, et al. Natural history of hepatitis D viral superinfection: significance of viremia detected by polymerase chain reaction. Gastroenterology. 1995;108(3):796–802.
36. Rizzetto M, Verme G, Recchia S, et al. Chronic hepatitis in carriers of hepatitis B surface antigen, with intrahepatic expression of the delta antigen. An active and progressive disease unresponsive to immunosuppressive treatment. Ann Intern Med. 1983;98(4):437–441.
37. Gheorghe L, Iacob S, Simionov I, et al. Natural history of compensated viral B and D cirrhosis. Rom J Gastroenterol. 2005;14(4):329–335.
38. Romeo R, Del Ninno E, Rumi M, et al. A 28-year study of the course of hepatitis Delta infection: a risk factor for cirrhosis and hepatocellular carcinoma. Gastroenterology. 2009;136(5): 1629–1638.
39. Su CW, Huang YH, Huo TI, et al. Genotypes and viremia of hepatitis B and D viruses are associated with outcomes of chronic hepatitis D patients. Gastroenterology. 2006;130(6):1625–1635.
40. Castellares C, Barreiro P, Martin-Carbonero L, et al. Liver cirrhosis in HIV-infected patients: prevalence, aetiology and clinical outcome. J Viral Hepat. 2008;15(3):165–172.
41. Sheng WH, Hung CC, Kao JH, et al. Impact of hepatitis D virus infection on the long-term outcomes of patients with hepatitis B virus and HIV coinfection in the era of highly active antiretroviral therapy: a matched cohort study. Clin Infect Dis. 2007;44(7):988–995.
42. Wu JC, Choo KB, Chen CM, Chen TZ, Huo TI, Lee SD. Genotyping of hepatitis D virus by restriction-fragment length polymorphism and relation to outcome of hepatitis D. Lancet. 1995;346(8980):939–941.
43. Casey JL, Brown TL, Colan EJ, Wignall FS, Gerin JL. A genotype of hepatitis D virus that occurs in northern South America. Proc Natl Acad Sci U S A. 1993;90(19):9016–9020.
44. Bensabath G, Hadler SC, Soares MC, et al. Hepatitis delta virus infection and Labrea hepatitis. Prevalence and role in fulminant hepatitis in the Amazon Basin. JAMA. 1987;258(4): 479–483.
45. Hadler SC, Alcala de Monzon M, Rivero D, Perez M, Bracho A, Fields H. Epidemiology and long-term consequences of hepatitis delta virus infection in the Yucpa Indians of Venezuela. Am J Epidemiol. 1992;136(12):1507–1516.
46. Shih HH, Jeng KS, Syu WJ, et al. Hepatitis B surface antigen levels and sequences of natural hepatitis B virus variants influence the assembly and secretion of hepatitis d virus. J Virol. 2008;82(5):2250–2264.
47. Farci P, Barbera C, Navone C, et al. Infection with the delta agent in children. Gut. 1985; 26(1):4–7.
48. Zuckerman AJ. Prevention of primary liver cancer by immunization. N Engl J Med. 1997;336(26): 1906–1907.
49. Borresen ML, Olsen OR, Ladefoged K, et al. Hepatitis D outbreak among children in a hepatitis B hyper-endemic settlement in Greenland. J Viral Hepat. 2010;17:162–170.
50. Morcos MM, Mikhail TH, Hanna WM, Abdel-Fattah S, el-Rasad MM, Wassef EL. The prevalence of delta virus infection in chronic liver disease in Egyptian children in comparison with some other countries. Panminerva Med. 2000;42(2):97–100.
51. Zanetti AR, Ferroni P, Magliano EM, et al. Perinatal transmission of the hepatitis B virus and of the HBV-associated delta agent from mothers to offspring in northern Italy. J Med Virol. 1982;9(2):139–148.
52. Bichko V, Netter HJ, Wu TT, Taylor J. Pathogenesis associated with replication of hepatitis delta virus. Infect Agents Dis. 1994;3(2–3):94–97.

53. Nakano T, Shapiro CN, Hadler SC, et al. Characterization of hepatitis D virus genotype III among Yucpa Indians in Venezuela. J Gen Virol. 2001;82(Pt 9):2183–2189.
54. Zachou K, Yurdaydin C, Drebber U, et al. Quantitative HBsAg and HDV-RNA levels in chronic delta hepatitis. Liver Internat. 2009.
55. Zachou K, Yurdaydin C, Dienes HE, Dalekos GN, Erhardt A, Cakaloglu Y, Degertekin H, Gurel S, Zeuzem S, Bozkaya H, Bock T, Schlaphoff V, Manns MP, Wedemeyer H. 479 Significance of HDV-RNA and HBsAg levels in delta hepatitis: first data of the Hep-Net/international HDV intervention trial. J Hepatol. 2006;44:S178.
56. Aragona M, Macagno S, Caredda F, et al. Serological response to the hepatitis delta virus in hepatitis D. Lancet. 1987;1(8531):478–480.
57. Govindarajan S, Valinluck B, Peters L. Relapse of acute B viral hepatitis – role of delta agent. Gut. 1986;27(1):19–22.
58. Shattock AG, Morgan BM. Sensitive enzyme immunoassay for the detection of delta antigen and anti-delta, using serum as the delta antigen source. J Med Virol. 1984;13(1):73–82.
59. Wedemeyer H, Manns MP. Epidemiology, pathogenesis and management of hepatitis D: update and challenges ahead. Nat Rev Gastroenterol Hepatol. 2010;7(1):31–40.
60. Parana R, Kay A, Molinet F, et al. HDV genotypes in the Western Brazilian Amazon region: a preliminary report. Am J Trop Med Hyg. 2006;75(3):475–479.
61. Buti M, Esteban R, Jardi R, Esteban JI, Guardia J. Serological diagnosis of acute delta hepatitis. J Med Virol. 1986;18(1):81–85.
62. Smedile A, Lavarini C, Crivelli O, Raimondo G, Fassone M, Rizzetto M. Radioimmunoassay detection of IgM antibodies to the HBV-associated delta (delta) antigen: clinical significance in delta infection. J Med Virol. 1982;9(2):131–138.
63. Zignego AL, Deny P, Feray C, et al. Amplification of hepatitis delta virus RNA sequences by polymerase chain reaction: a tool for viral detection and cloning. Mol Cell Probes. 1990;4(1):43–51.
64. Madejon A, Castillo I, Bartolome J, et al. Detection of HDV-RNA by PCR in serum of patients with chronic HDV infection. J Hepatol. 1990;11(3):381–384.
65. Dinolfo L, Abate ML, Bertolo P, et al. Detection of hepatitis D virus RNA in serum by a reverse transcription, polymerase chain reaction-based assay. Int J Clin Lab Res. 1995;25(1):35–39.
66. McFarlane IG, Chaggar K, Davies SE, Smith HM, Alexander GJ, Williams R. IgA class antibodies to hepatitis delta virus antigen in acute and chronic hepatitis delta virus infections. Hepatology. 1991;14(6):980–984.
67. Rizzetto M, Rosina F, Saracco G, et al. Treatment of chronic delta hepatitis with alpha-2 recombinant interferon. J Hepatol. 1986;3 Suppl 2:S229–S233.
68. Ilan Y, Klein A, Taylor J, Tur-Kaspa R. Resistance of hepatitis delta virus replication to interferon-alpha treatment in transfected human cells. J Infect Dis. 1992;166(5):1164–1166.
69. McNair AN, Cheng D, Monjardino J, Thomas HC, Kerr IM. Hepatitis delta virus replication in vitro is not affected by interferon-alpha or -gamma despite intact cellular responses to interferon and dsRNA. J Gen Virol. 1994;75 (Pt 6):1371–1378.
70. Farci P, Mandas A, Coiana A, et al. Treatment of chronic hepatitis D with interferon alfa-2a. N Engl J Med. 1994;330(2):88–94.
71. Farci P, Roskams T, Chessa L, et al. Long-term benefit of interferon alpha therapy of chronic hepatitis D: regression of advanced hepatic fibrosis. Gastroenterology. 2004;126(7): 1740–1749.
72. Niro GA, Rosina F, Rizzetto M. Treatment of hepatitis D. J Viral Hepat. 2005;12(1):2–9.
73. Yurdaydin C, Bozkaya H, Karaaslan H, et al. A pilot study of 2 years of interferon treatment in patients with chronic delta hepatitis. J Viral Hepat. 2007;14(11):812–816.
74. Castelnau C, Le Gal F, Ripault MP, et al. Efficacy of peginterferon alpha-2b in chronic hepatitis delta: relevance of quantitative RT-PCR for follow-up. Hepatology. 2006;44(3):728–735.
75. Erhardt A, Gerlich W, Starke C, et al. Treatment of chronic hepatitis delta with pegylated interferon-alpha2b. Liver Internat. 2006;26(7):805–810.

76. Niro GA, Ciancio A, Gaeta GB, et al. Pegylated interferon alpha-2b as monotherapy or in combination with ribavirin in chronic hepatitis delta. Hepatology. 2006;44(3):713–720.
77. Yurdaydin C, Wedemeyer H, Dalekos G, et al. A multicenter randomised stduy comparing the efficacy of pegylated intereron alfa-2A plus adefovir dipivoxil vs. pegylated intereron alfa-2A plus placebo vs. adefovir dipovoxil for the treatment of chronic delta hepatitis: the intervention trial (HID-IT). Hepatology 2006;41(suppl 1):230A.
78. Niro GA, Ciancio A, Tillman HL, et al. Lamivudine therapy in chronic delta hepatitis: a multicentre randomized-controlled pilot study. Aliment Pharmacol Ther. 2005;22(3):227–232.
79. Wolters LM, van Nunen AB, Honkoop P, et al. Lamivudine-high dose interferon combination therapy for chronic hepatitis B patients co-infected with the hepatitis D virus. J Viral Hepat. 2000;7(6):428–434.
80. Lau DT, Doo E, Park Y, et al. Lamivudine for chronic delta hepatitis. Hepatology. 1999;30(2):546–549.
81. Gunsar F, Akarca US, Ersoz G, et al. Two-year interferon therapy with or without ribavirin in chronic delta hepatitis. Antivir Ther. 2005;10(6):721–726.
82. Garripoli A, Di Marco V, Cozzolongo R, et al. Ribavirin treatment for chronic hepatitis D: a pilot study. Liver. 1994;14(3):154–157.
83. Schneider A, Habermehl P, Gerner P, Lausch E, Ballauff A, Wirth S. Alpha-interferon treatment in HBeAg positive children with chronic hepatitis B and associated hepatitis D. Klin Padiatr. 1998;210(5):363–365.
84. Dalekos GN, Galanakis E, Zervou E, Tzoufi M, Lapatsanis PD, Tsianos EV. Interferon-alpha treatment of children with chronic hepatitis D virus infection: the Greek experience. Hepatogastroenterology. 2000;47(34):1072–1076.
85. Samuel D, Muller R, Alexander G, et al. Liver transplantation in European patients with the hepatitis B surface antigen. N Engl J Med. 1993;329(25):1842–1847.
86. Balayan MS, Andjaparidze AG, Savinskaya SS, et al. Evidence for a virus in non-A, non-B hepatitis transmitted via the fecal-oral route. Intervirology. 1983;20(1):23–31.
87. Reyes GR, Purdy MA, Kim JP, et al. Isolation of a cDNA from the virus responsible for enterically transmitted non-A, non-B hepatitis. Science. 1990;247(4948):1335–1339.
88. Tsarev SA, Emerson SU, Reyes GR, et al. Characterization of a prototype strain of hepatitis E virus. Proc Natl Acad Sci U S A. 1992;89(2):559–563.
89. Tam AW, Smith MM, Guerra ME, et al. Hepatitis E virus (HEV): molecular cloning and sequencing of the full-length viral genome. Virology. 1991;185(1):120–131.
90. Ansari IH, Nanda SK, Durgapal H, et al. Cloning, sequencing, and expression of the hepatitis E virus (HEV) nonstructural open reading frame 1 (ORF1). J Med Virol. 2000;60(3):275–283.
91. Krawczynski K, Bradley DW. Enterically transmitted non-A, non-B hepatitis: identification of virus-associated antigen in experimentally infected cynomolgus macaques. J Infect Dis. 1989;159(6):1042–1049.
92. Worm HC, van der Poel WH, Brandstatter G. Hepatitis E: an overview. Microbes Infect. 2002;4(6):657–666.
93. Aggarwal R, Krawczynski K. Hepatitis E: an overview and recent advances in clinical and laboratory research. J Gastroenterol Hepatol. 2000;15(1):9–20.
94. Lu L, Li C, Hagedorn CH. Phylogenetic analysis of global hepatitis E virus sequences: genetic diversity, subtypes and zoonosis. Rev Med Virol. 2006;16(1):5–36.
95. Huang CC, Nguyen D, Fernandez J, et al. Molecular cloning and sequencing of the Mexico isolate of hepatitis E virus (HEV). Virology. 1992;191(2):550–558.
96. van Cuyck-Gandre H, Zhang HY, Tsarev SA, et al. Characterization of hepatitis E virus (HEV) from Algeria and Chad by partial genome sequence. J Med Virol. 1997;53(4):340–347.
97. Dalton HR, Bendall R, Ijaz S, Banks M. Hepatitis E: an emerging infection in developed countries. Lancet Infect Dis. 2008;8(11):698–709.

98. Wang Y, Ling R, Erker JC, et al. A divergent genotype of hepatitis E virus in Chinese patients with acute hepatitis. J Gen Virol. 1999;80 (Pt 1):169–177.
99. Naik SR, Aggarwal R, Salunke PN, Mehrotra NN. A large waterborne viral hepatitis E epidemic in Kanpur, India. Bull World Health Organ. 1992;70(5):597–604.
100. Khuroo MS. Study of an epidemic of non-A, non-B hepatitis. Possibility of another human hepatitis virus distinct from post-transfusion non-A, non-B type. Am J Med. 1980;68(6):818–824.
101. Kane MA, Bradley DW, Shrestha SM, et al. Epidemic non-A, non-B hepatitis in Nepal. Recovery of a possible etiologic agent and transmission studies in marmosets. JAMA. 1984;252(22):3140–3145.
102. Tsega E, Hansson BG, Krawczynski K, Nordenfelt E. Acute sporadic viral hepatitis in Ethiopia: causes, risk factors, and effects on pregnancy. Clin Infect Dis. 1992;14(4): 961–965.
103. Aggarwal R, Shahi H, Naik S, Yachha SK, Naik SR. Evidence in favour of high infection rate with hepatitis E virus among young children in India. J Hepatol. 1997;26(6):1425–1426.
104. Aggarwal R, Naik SR. Hepatitis E: does person-to-person spread occur? Indian J Gastroenterol. 1992;11(3):109–112.
105. Somani SK, Aggarwal R, Naik SR, Srivastava S, Naik S. A serological study of intrafamilial spread from patients with sporadic hepatitis E virus infection. J Viral Hepat. 2003;10(6): 446–449.
106. Khuroo MS, Kamili S, Yattoo GN. Hepatitis E virus infection may be transmitted through blood transfusions in an endemic area. J Gastroenterol Hepatol. 2004;19(7):778–784.
107. Arankalle VA, Chobe LP. Retrospective analysis of blood transfusion recipients: evidence for post-transfusion hepatitis E. Vox Sang. 2000;79(2):72–74.
108. Matsubayashi K, Nagaoka Y, Sakata H, et al. Transfusion-transmitted hepatitis E caused by apparently indigenous hepatitis E virus strain in Hokkaido, Japan. Transfusion. 2004;44(6): 934–940.
109. Singh S, Mohanty A, Joshi YK, Deka D, Mohanty S, Panda SK. Mother-to-child transmission of hepatitis E virus infection. Indian J Pediatr. 2003;70(1):37–39.
110. Velazquez O, Stetler HC, Avila C, et al. Epidemic transmission of enterically transmitted non-A, non-B hepatitis in Mexico, 1986–1987. JAMA. 1990;263(24):3281–3285.
111. Belabbes EH, Bouguermouh A, Benatallah A, Illoul G. Epidemic non-A, non-B viral hepatitis in Algeria: strong evidence for its spreading by water. J Med Virol. 1985;16(3):257–263.
112. Tsega E, Krawczynski K, Hansson BG, et al. Outbreak of acute hepatitis E virus infection among military personnel in northern Ethiopia. J Med Virol. 1991;34(4):232–236.
113. Nicand E, Armstrong GL, Enouf V, et al. Genetic heterogeneity of hepatitis E virus in Darfur, Sudan, and neighboring Chad. J Med Virol. 2005;77(4):519–521.
114. Meng XJ. Hepatitis E virus: animal reservoirs and zoonotic risk. Vet Microbiol. 2009;140(3–4): 256–265.
115. Tei S, Kitajima N, Takahashi K, Mishiro S. Zoonotic transmission of hepatitis E virus from deer to human beings. Lancet. 2003;362(9381):371–373.
116. Li TC, Chijiwa K, Sera N, et al. Hepatitis E virus transmission from wild boar meat. Emerg Infect Dis. 2005;11(12):1958–1960.
117. Wichmann O, Schimanski S, Koch J, et al. Phylogenetic and case-control study on hepatitis E virus infection in Germany. J Infect Dis. 2008;198(12):1732–1741.
118. Meng XJ, Wiseman B, Elvinger F, et al. Prevalence of antibodies to hepatitis E virus in veterinarians working with swine and in normal blood donors in the United States and other countries. J Clin Microbiol. 2002;40(1):117–122.
119. Banks M, Bendall R, Grierson S, Heath G, Mitchell J, Dalton H. Human and porcine hepatitis E virus strains, United Kingdom. Emerg Infect Dis. 2004;10(5):953–955.
120. Karetnyi YV, Gilchrist MJ, Naides SJ. Hepatitis E virus infection prevalence among selected populations in Iowa. J Clin Virol. 1999;14(1):51–55.
121. Kuniholm MH, Purcell RH, McQuillan GM, Engle RE, Wasley A, Nelson KE. Epidemiology of hepatitis E virus in the United States: results from the Third National Health and Nutrition Examination Survey, 1988–1994. J Infect Dis. 2009;200(1):48–56.

122. Khuroo MS, Kamili S, Jameel S. Vertical transmission of hepatitis E virus. Lancet. 1995;345(8956):1025–1026.
123. Kumar RM, Uduman S, Rana S, Kochiyil JK, Usmani A, Thomas L. Sero-prevalence and mother-to-infant transmission of hepatitis E virus among pregnant women in the United Arab Emirates. Eur J Obstet Gynecol Reprod Biol. 2001;100(1):9–15.
124. Chau TN, Lai ST, Tse C, et al. Epidemiology and clinical features of sporadic hepatitis E as compared with hepatitis A. Am J Gastroenterol. 2006;101(2):292–296.
125. Khuroo MS, Teli MR, Skidmore S, Sofi MA, Khuroo MI. Incidence and severity of viral hepatitis in pregnancy. Am J Med. 1981;70(2):252–255.
126. Hamid SS, Atiq M, Shehzad F, et al. Hepatitis E virus superinfection in patients with chronic liver disease. Hepatology. 2002;36(2):474–478.
127. Kumar Acharya S, Kumar Sharma P, Singh R, et al. Hepatitis E virus (HEV) infection in patients with cirrhosis is associated with rapid decompensation and death. J Hepatol. 2007;46(3):387–394.
128. Haagsma EB, van den Berg AP, Porte RJ, et al. Chronic hepatitis E virus infection in liver transplant recipients. Liver Transpl. 2008;14(4):547–553.
129. Kamar N, Selves J, Mansuy JM, et al. Hepatitis E virus and chronic hepatitis in organ-transplant recipients. N Engl J Med. 2008;358(8):811–817.
130. Ollier L, Tieulie N, Sanderson F, et al. Chronic hepatitis after hepatitis E virus infection in a patient with non-Hodgkin lymphoma taking rituximab. Ann Intern Med. 2009;150(6):430–431.
131. Chauhan A, Jameel S, Dilawari JB, Chawla YK, Kaur U, Ganguly NK. Hepatitis E virus transmission to a volunteer. Lancet. 1993;341(8838):149–150.
132. Favorov MO, Fields HA, Purdy MA, et al. Serologic identification of hepatitis E virus infections in epidemic and endemic settings. J Med Virol. 1992;36(4):246–250.
133. Arora NK, Panda SK, Nanda SK, et al. Hepatitis E infection in children: study of an outbreak. J Gastroenterol Hepatol. 1999;14(6):572–577.
134. de Groen PC. Hepatitis E in the United States: a case of "hog fever"? Mayo Clin Proc. 1997;72(12):1197–1198.
135. Kar P, Jilani N, Husain SA, et al. Does hepatitis E viral load and genotypes influence the final outcome of acute liver failure during pregnancy? Am J Gastroenterol. 2008;103(10):2495–2501.
136. Patra S, Kumar A, Trivedi SS, Puri M, Sarin SK. Maternal and fetal outcomes in pregnant women with acute hepatitis E virus infection. Ann Intern Med. 2007;147(1):28–33.
137. Bhatia V, Singhal A, Panda SK, Acharya SK. A 20-year single-center experience with acute liver failure during pregnancy: is the prognosis really worse? Hepatology. 2008;48(5):1577–1585.
138. Gerolami R, Moal V, Colson P. Chronic hepatitis E with cirrhosis in a kidney-transplant recipient. N Engl J Med. 2008;358(8):859–860.
139. Dalton HR, Bendall RP, Keane FE, Tedder RS, Ijaz S. Persistent carriage of hepatitis E virus in patients with HIV infection. N Engl J Med. 2009;361(10):1025–1027.
140. Soe S, Uchida T, Suzuki K, et al. Enterically transmitted non-A, non-B hepatitis in cynomolgus monkeys: morphology and probable mechanism of hepatocellular necrosis. Liver. 1989;9(3):135–145.
141. Gupta DN, Smetana HF. The histopathology of viral hepatitis as seen in the Delhi epidemic (1955–56). Indian J Med Res. 1957;45(Suppl.):101–113.
142. Asher LV, Innis BL, Shrestha MP, Ticehurst J, Baze WB. Virus-like particles in the liver of a patient with fulminant hepatitis and antibody to hepatitis E virus. J Med Virol. 1990;31(3):229–233.
143. Clayson ET, Myint KS, Snitbhan R, et al. Viremia, fecal shedding, and IgM and IgG responses in patients with hepatitis E. J Infect Dis. 1995;172(4):927–933.
144. Bryan JP, Tsarev SA, Iqbal M, et al. Epidemic hepatitis E in Pakistan: patterns of serologic response and evidence that antibody to hepatitis E virus protects against disease. J Infect Dis. 1994;170(3):517–521.

145. Favorov MO, Khudyakov YE, Mast EE, et al. IgM and IgG antibodies to hepatitis E virus (HEV) detected by an enzyme immunoassay based on an HEV-specific artificial recombinant mosaic protein. J Med Virol. 1996;50(1):50–58.
146. Gyarmati P, Mohammed N, Norder H, Blomberg J, Belak S, Widen F. Universal detection of hepatitis E virus by two real-time PCR assays: TaqMan and Primer-Probe Energy Transfer. J Virol Methods. 2007;146(1–2):226–235.
147. Joshi YK, Babu S, Sarin S, Tandon BN, Gandhi BM, Chaturvedi VC. Immunoprophylaxis of epidemic non-A non-B hepatitis. Indian J Med Res. 1985;81:18–19.
148. Khuroo MS, Dar MY. Hepatitis E: evidence for person-to-person transmission and inability of low dose immune serum globulin from an Indian source to prevent it. Indian J Gastroenterol. 1992;11(3):113–116.
149. Tsarev SA, Tsareva TS, Emerson SU, et al. Successful passive and active immunization of cynomolgus monkeys against hepatitis E. Proc Natl Acad Sci U S A. 1994;91(21):10198–10202.
150. Bile K, Isse A, Mohamud O, et al. Contrasting roles of rivers and wells as sources of drinking water on attack and fatality rates in a hepatitis E epidemic in Somalia. Am J Trop Med Hyg. 1994;51(4):466–474.
151. Corwin AL, Khiem HB, Clayson ET, et al. A waterborne outbreak of hepatitis E virus transmission in southwestern Vietnam. Am J Trop Med Hyg. 1996;54(6):559–562.
152. Aggarwal R, Naik SR. Hepatitis E: intrafamilial transmission versus waterborne spread. J Hepatol. 1994;21(5):718–723.
153. Khuroo MS. Hepatitis E: the enterically transmitted non-A, non-B hepatitis. Indian J Gastroenterol. 1991;10(3):96–100.
154. Hong Y, Ruan B, Yang LH, et al. Hepatitis E virus chimeric DNA vaccine elicits immunologic response in mice. World J Gastroenterol. 2005;11(42):6713–6715.
155. Zhang M, Emerson SU, Nguyen H, et al. Recombinant vaccine against hepatitis E: duration of protective immunity in rhesus macaques. Vaccine. 2002;20(27–28):3285–3291.
156. Purcell RH, Nguyen H, Shapiro M, et al. Pre-clinical immunogenicity and efficacy trial of a recombinant hepatitis E vaccine. Vaccine. 2003;21(19–20):2607–2615.
157. Zhou YX, Lee MY, Ng JM, et al. A truncated hepatitis E virus ORF2 protein expressed in tobacco plastids is immunogenic in mice. World J Gastroenterol. 2006;12(2):306–312.
158. Shrestha MP, Scott RM, Joshi DM, et al. Safety and efficacy of a recombinant hepatitis E vaccine. N Engl J Med. 2007;356(9):895–903.
159. Zhang J, Liu CB, Li RC, et al. Randomized-controlled phase II clinical trial of a bacterially expressed recombinant hepatitis E vaccine. Vaccine. 2009;27(12):1869–1874.
160. Aggarwal R, Naik S. Epidemiology of hepatitis E: current status. J Gastroenterol Hepatol. 2009;24(9):1484–1493.

Hepatitis in Children due to Non-A–E Viruses

Karan Emerick

Key Concepts

- Neonatal hepatitis is a descriptive term that refers to the changes seen in the liver of neonates with many different viral infections.
- For congenital viral infections, the gestational age at which the infection occurs is critically important in determining the incidence of associated malformations.
- The clinical manifestations and prognosis of non-A through E viral hepatitis infections are largely determined by factors related to the host such as age and immunocompetence at the time of infection.
- The Herpesvirus family can produce a wide variety of liver diseases with particular susceptibility in the immunocompromised host (such as the neonate or transplanted patient), leading to risk of hepatic failure. Some of the viruses in this family include CMV, EBV, HSV, and HHV-6.
- In the susceptible host, such as the neonate, serious disseminated viral disease may be very nonspecific in presentation but have a high morbidity if not treated quickly. Severe hepatitis with systemic symptoms in the neonate requires rapid evaluation and possibly pre-emptive antiviral therapy.

Keywords Congenital viral infection • Cytomegalovirus • Epstein–Barr virus • Herpes simplex virus • Human herpesvirus 6 • Rubella • Enterovirus • Parvovirus • Paramxyovirus • Human immunodeficiency virus • Neonatal hepatitis • Congenital viral infection • Neonatal liver failure • Hepatic fibrosis • Granulomatous hepatitis • Intravenous immunoglobulin • Neonatal liver transplantation • Acyclovir • Ganciclovir • Pleconaril

K. Emerick (✉)
Pediatric Digestive Diseases, Connecticut Children's Medical Center,
282 Washington Street, Hartford, CT 06106, USA
e-mail: Kemerick@ccmckids.org

M.M. Jonas (ed.), *Viral Hepatitis in Children: Unique Features and Opportunities*,
Clinical Gastroenterology, DOI 10.1007/978-1-60761-373-2_7,

Introduction

Viral infections that primarily affect the liver such as hepatitis A through E are the cause of tremendous morbidity worldwide and have been described in the preceding chapters. Numerous other viruses primarily cause systemic disease but are also associated with hepatitis. The majority of these viruses result in a generalized illness or a constellation of symptoms that are multi-systemic. The liver can be involved to varying degrees depending on the mode of transmission and age at infection. This chapter will describe the patterns of disease associated with these viruses. These viruses include cytomegalovirus (CMV), Epstein–Barr virus (EBV), herpes simplex virus (HSV), human herpes virus 6 (HHV-6), rubella, enterovirus, parvovirus, paramyxovirus, and human immunodeficiency virus (HIV). The clinical manifestations and prognosis of these viral infections are largely determined by factors related to the host such as age and immunocompetence at the time of infection. Congenital infections will also be covered briefly.

Congenital Viral Infections

Many non-A–E viral infections not only cause hepatitis but also have been implicated in causing congenital malformations. These include rubella, cytomegalovirus, herpes simplex, varicella zoster, influenza, mumps, enterovirus, and HIV. Rubella virus and CMV are the most common. The gestational age at which the infection occurs in the mother is critically important in both cases.

The highest risk period for rubella infection extends from before conception to the sixteenth week of gestation. The incidence of malformations is reduced from >80% to 20% to 7% if infection occurs in the first, second, or third month of gestation [1]. The fetal defects are varied, but the major tetrad comprises cataracts, heart defects (persistent ductus arteriosus, pulmonary artery hypoplasia or stenosis, ventricular septal defect, and tetralogy of Fallot), deafness, and mental retardation, referred to as congenital rubella syndrome [1].

CMV is the most common fetal viral infection and, although associated with congenital anomalies, it mostly causes asymptomatic infection [1, 2]. The risk of congenital abnormalities is the highest with intrauterine CMV infection in the second trimester of pregnancy [3, 4]. The vertical transmission rate has been recorded as 1–2% in populations with high maternal CMV seropositivity rate (95.7%) and 0.5–2.0% of all live births [4]. In general, factors associated with seropositivity include lower socioeconomic status, maternal age >30 years, less than a college education, and contact with young children. Clinical manifestations of infection are apparent in 5–10% of infants [5, 6]. These include intrauterine growth restriction, microcephaly, periventricular cerebral calcifications, thrombocytopenia, purpura, deafness, chorioretinitis, hyperbilirubinemia, and hepatosplenomegaly [6]. In addition, mental retardation, visual impairment, seizures, and developmental delay have all been described in congenital CMV. Mean values of viral blood load determined by quantitative polymerase chain reaction (PCR) are significantly higher in symptomatic newborns [3].

Neonatal Hepatitis

Neonatal hepatitis refers to hepatitis seen in the first months of life, usually secondary to a viral infection. Although hepatitis A–E viral infections do occur in neonates, other viruses are the main cause of disease. These include CMV, rubella, herpes simplex, HHV-6, coxsackievirus, echovirus, parvovirus B19, enteroviruses, and paramyxovirus (Table 1). A histological pattern of syncytial giant cell transformation and cholestasis is the common finding (Fig. 1). Giant cell hepatitis in the neonate may result in fulminant liver failure with massive hepatocyte necrosis, and the severe liver dysfunction may lead to death or the need for liver transplantation. However, the majority of cases will culminate in slow recovery [7–10]. The risk of liver failure relates to the particular virus as discussed below.

The Herpesvirus Family

The Herpesvirus family can produce a wide variety of liver diseases with particular susceptibility in the immunocompromised host. Some of the viruses in this family include CMV, EBV, HSV, and HHV-6. Herpesviruses persist life-long in a latent non-replicative state after resolution of the primary infection [11].

Cytomegalovirus

Cytomegalovirus (CMV) is a double-stranded DNA virus that is endemic in the human population. It not only can cause significant pathology in immunodeficient patients but may also cause disease in individuals with normal immune systems. Acute anicteric hepatitis, as a part of systemic mononucleosis-type illness, is the most common presentation in a healthy host. The CMV virus replicates in both hepatocytes and cholangiocytes during infection; therefore, the spectrum of disease ranges from mild aminotransferase elevation to cholestatic hepatitis to hepatic necrosis. Besides being the most common cause of congenital viral infection in the USA, approximately 20% of children less than 15 years of age and 50–60% of individuals younger than 25–30 years of age are infected with CMV [5]. CMV has been isolated from oropharyngeal secretions, urine, feces, semen, breast milk, blood, and tears. In neonates CMV infection may be acquired transplacentally, during delivery, or postnatally from body fluids such as saliva and breast milk [12]. In adults and children, transmission is by close personal contact.

Table 1 Systemic viral infections that involve the liver, their associated clinical and hepatic histologic findings, means of diagnosis and potential treatment

Virus	Liver findings	Diagnosis	Treatment
CMV	Giant cell hepatitis Intranuclear inclusion bodies in bile duct epithelium or intracytoplasmic inclusion bodies in hepatocytes	Viral culture: urine, saliva, nasopharyngeal secretions, and blood CMV PCR from blood Tissue staining with monoclonal antibodies Serology	Ganciclovir CMV immunoglobulin
EBV	Atypical lymphocytes in the portal areas and sinusoids, scattered Isolated foci of parenchymal necrosis	EBV PCR from blood or tissue Serology	Acyclovir
Herpes	Giant cell hepatitis necrosis	HSV PCR from blood DFA of lesion Immunostaining of tissue	Acyclovir
HHV-6	Giant cell hepatitis Hepatocellular necrosis	PCR of tissue or blood	
Rubella	Giant cell hepatitis Mononuclear infiltrate of portal zone with fibrosis Cholestasis	Culture of throat swabs, urine, blood or CSF Serology PCR (research)	Supportive
Enterovirus	Hepatic necrosis	Culture of throat swabs or, rectum or biopsy material PCR (experimental)	Pleconaril IVIG
Parvovirus	Giant cell hepatitis	B19 Parvovirus IgM antibody from blood PCR	Monoclonal anti-CD52 antibodies IVIG
Paramyxovirus	Giant cell hepatitis Bridging necrosis Cholestasis	Histological identification of viral structure in tissue	Supportive
Human immunodeficiency virus	Giant cell hepatitis Granulomatous hepatitis	HIV ELISA or Western blot HIV PCR	Antiretroviral therapy

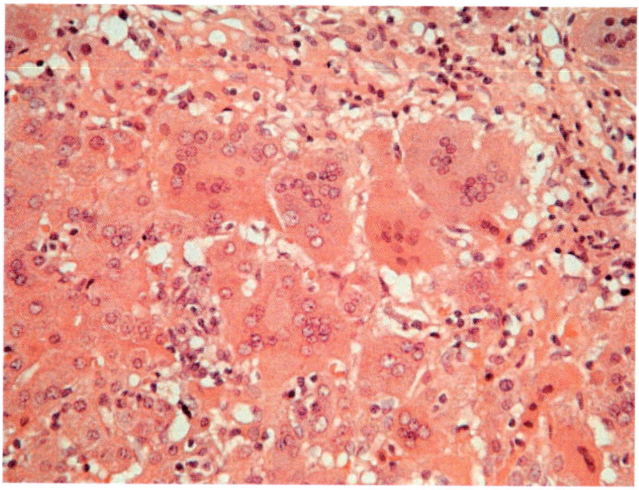

Fig. 1 Pathological findings of neonatal hepatitis with multinucleated giant cells. H&E

In congenital CMV infection, neonatal hepatosplenomegaly is the usual finding. Mild hepatitis and elevated bilirubin levels may also occur. The histological appearance of the infected liver may show significant giant cell transformation, lymphomonocytic cell infiltration, hydropic degeneration, mild steatosis, perisinusoidal fibrosis, Kupffer cell hyperplasia, large intranuclear inclusion bodies in bile duct epithelium, or intracytoplasmic inclusion bodies in hepatocytes [13]. The infected neonatal liver will also usually show evidence of extramedullary hematopoiesis and round cell infiltration of the portal tracts [5]. In children infected after birth, both inclusion bodies and microabcesses consisting of polymorphonuclear leukocytes in the hepatic parenchyma can be seen (Fig. 2). Infants with congenital CMV may appear to resolve their acute inflammatory process over time and yet may go on to develop portal hypertension with diffuse hepatic fibrosis [14, 15].

CMV infection can present with a life-threatening multi-organ process in immunosuppressed patients. This would include posttransplant patients and patients with rheumatologic diseases. CMV is the second most common viral infection in patients with systemic lupus erythematosus and, in this setting, infection may mimic a lupus flare or present with specific organ involvement such as hepatitis, gastrointestinal bleeding, or pulmonary infiltrates.

The diagnosis of CMV infection may be made from viral culture of body fluids (urine, nasopharyngeal secretions or saliva, and blood). Virus can also be detected by PCR testing of blood for viral DNA or staining tissue with monoclonal antibodies for CMV. Serologies for CMV IgG and IgM can clarify previous versus current infection. Immunocompromised patients (i.e., HIV+ and solid-organ recipients) may develop reactivation of latent infection and in these cases, the "shell viral " assay (monoclonal antibodies used to detect CMV antigens) or using assays such as the pp65 antigenemia assay may be helpful because antigenemia precedes organ

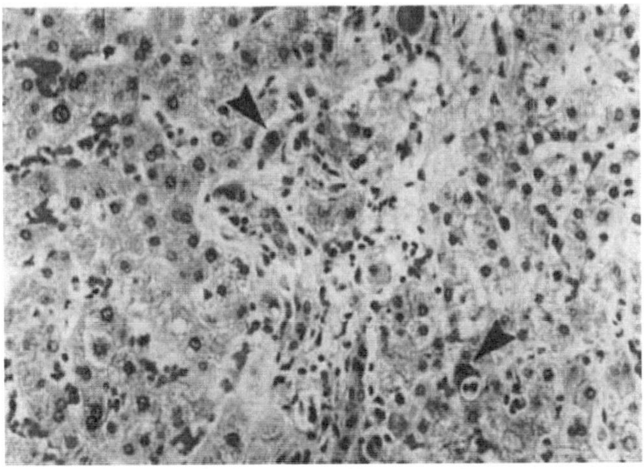

Fig. 2 Pathological findings in cytomegalovirus hepatitis. Large, intranuclear inclusion in hepatocyte shown by arrow. (From *Schneiderman DJ, et al, Hepatic disease in patients with the acquired immune deficiency syndrome (AIDS). Hepatology, Dec 7, 2005, p. 925*)

involvement. Antiviral treatment for CMV is usually ganciclovir alone or in conjunction with CMV immunoglobulin (CMVIG) infusions [13]. CMVIG is prepared from multiple donors who have high-titer CMV antibody levels (Table 1). Because it often takes months to develop the neutralizing antibody and high-avidity antibody to CMV, CMVIG theoretically provides high-avidity neutralizing antibody to rapidly combat the viremia. In a study of infants diagnosed with neonatal cytomegalovirus hepatitis, antiviral treatment with ganciclovir resulted in significant improvement of cholestatic and virologic markers, while the non-treated comparison group did not reveal any significant change [13]. For the most resistant cases or cases that have severe renal compromise, who therefore cannot receive ganciclovir, foscarnet is an alternate choice. In immunocompromised patients with symptoms, antiviral therapy is indicated until viremia is reduced or undetectable. In immunocompetent children, primary CMV infection is usually a mononucleosis-like illness which is self-limited and does not require treatment. However, should progressive multi-organ involvement (i.e., pneumonitis, colitis, and hepatitis) develop, then treatment would be indicated.

Epstein–Barr Virus

EBV is a member of the Herpesvirus family and is an enveloped DNA virus (Fig. 3b). In addition to infectious mononucleosis (defined as the triad of fever, pharyngitis, and lymphadenopathy), EBV has been etiologically linked to nasopharyngeal carcinoma, Burkitt lymphoma, and post-transplant lymphoproliferative disease in stem cell and solid-organ recipients [16]. Hepatic involvement is common

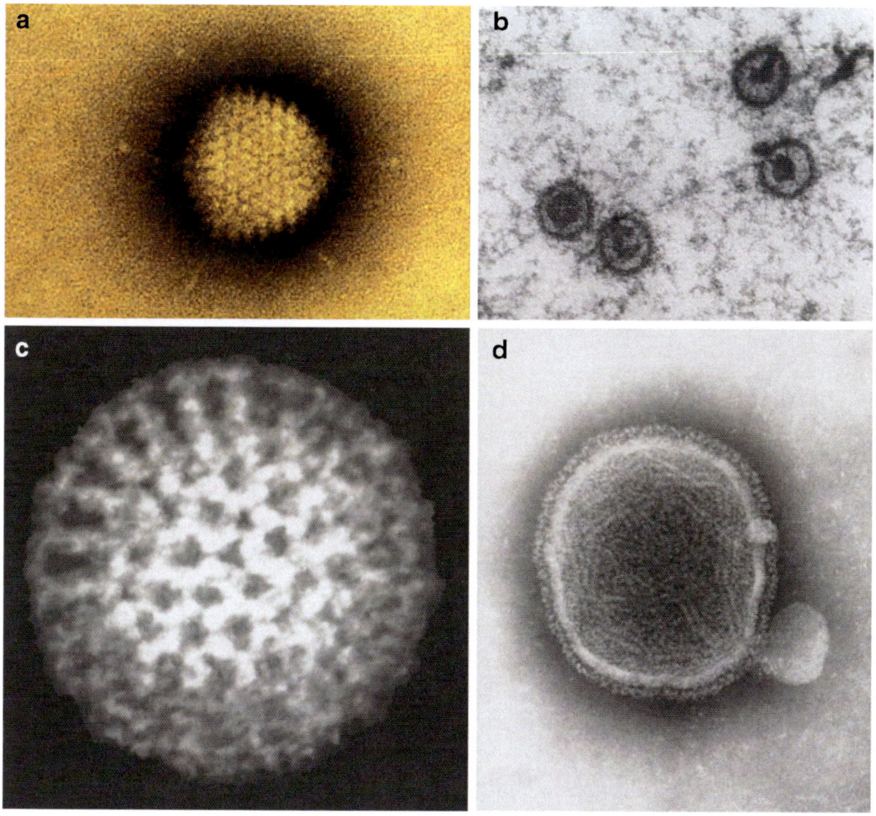

Fig. 3 Viral Structures seen by electron microscopy. (**a**) Adenovirus, an icosahedral nonenveloped DNA virus. (**b**) Epstein-Barr virus, an icosahedral envelope DNA virus. (**c**) Rotavirus, a nonenveloped, wheel-like, RNA virus. (**d**) Paramyxovirus, a spherical enveloped RNA virus. (From *Kumar: Robbins and Cotran Pathologic Basis of Diseases, Professional Edition, 8th ed. Figure 8-1*)

in EBV infection, and varies in severity. Like CMV, EBV infection can result in a range of liver diseases from mild self-resolving hepatitis to fatal hepatic necrosis.

EBV has a linear DNA molecule that encodes nearly 100 viral proteins. These proteins are important for regulating the expression of viral genes, replicating viral DNA, forming structural components of the virion, and modulating the host immune response. Infection of epithelial cells by EBV in vitro results in active replication, with production of virus and lysis of the cells [16]. In contrast, infection of B cells by EBV in vitro results in a latent infection, with immortalization of the cells.

EBV is one of the most successful viruses, infecting over 90% of humans and persisting for the lifetime of the person [16]. Infection of humans with EBV usually occurs by contact with oral secretions. The virus replicates in cells in the oropharynx, and nearly all seropositive persons actively shed virus in the saliva.

Whereas most EBV infections of infants and children are asymptomatic or have nonspecific symptoms, infections of adolescents and adults frequently result in infectious mononucleosis. Over 50% of patients with infectious mononucleosis manifest the triad of fever, lymphadenopathy, and pharyngitis; splenomegaly, palatal petechiae, and hepatomegaly are each present in more than 10% of patients. Less common complications include hemolytic anemia, thrombocytopenia, aplastic anemia, myocarditis, hepatitis, genital ulcers, splenic rupture, rash, and neurologic complications such as Guillain–Barré syndrome, encephalitis, and meningitis [16].

Most patients with infectious mononucleosis have leukocytosis with an absolute increase in peripheral mononuclear cells, heterophile antibodies, elevated serum aminotransferase levels, and atypical lymphocytes. The atypical lymphocytes are primary T cells, many of which respond to the EBV-infected B cells. Most of the symptoms of infectious mononucleosis are attributed to the proliferation and activation of T cells in response to infection. Up to a few percent of the peripheral B cells may be infected with EBV in infectious mononucleosis.

Chronic active EBV infection is a very rare disorder that has been defined by the following three features: severe illness of more than 6 months' duration that begins as a primary EBV infection or that is associated with abnormal EBV antibody titers; histologic evidence of organ disease, such as pneumonitis, hepatitis, bone marrow hypoplasia, or uveitis; and demonstration of EBV antigens or EBV DNA in tissue.

EBV liver involvement is usually mild, and resolves spontaneously [1]. Typically, the serum aminotransferase levels are mildly elevated. Severe cholestasis is rare. However, several case series have reported patients with documented acute EBV infection who have a primarily cholestatic pattern [17]. On histologic examination, atypical lymphocytes are seen in the portal areas and sinusoids, and scattered, isolated cells or foci of parenchymal necrosis may be present. This histologic picture is similar to that of other forms of acute viral hepatitis [17]. The diagnosis of EBV is usually based on the clinical findings, leukocytosis, and serologies. EBV infection is confirmed by the presence of serum concentrations of IgG and IgM antibodies against the EBV viral capsid antigen (anti-EBV VCA IgG), EBV early antigen, EBV nuclear antigen (EBV-EBNA), and heterophilic antibodies (monospot test). PCR assay of blood or tissue for EBV has become readily available and is a useful tool, particularly in immunocompromised patients. In immunocompetent patients with suspected primary infection, serology testing with EBV-specific immunoglobulin is adequate, whereas in immunocompromised patients, EBV PCR is more appropriate (Table 1).

No specific therapy is indicated for most patients with infectious mononucleosis. Although acyclovir inhibits EBV replication and reduces viral shedding, it has no significant effect on the symptoms of infectious mononucleosis (which are primarily due to the immune response to the virus) and is therefore not recommended [16]. Corticosteroids are generally not recommended for the treatment of uncomplicated disease, and should be considered for patients with severe complications of infectious mononucleosis, such as impending upper airway obstruction, acute hemolytic anemia, severe cardiac involvement, or neurologic disease. A double-blind, placebo-controlled study of combined therapy with acyclovir and prednisolone in uncomplicated infectious mononucleosis showed that this treatment did not affect the duration of illness or of absence from work [16]. In the immunocompromised patient or newborn with severe hepatitis, treatment with acyclovir will inhibit the replication of EBV and reduce viral shedding but may not alter the course of the illness.

Herpes Simplex Virus

Herpes Simplex Virus (HSV) infection is typically a mucocutaneous disease with lesions of the oral or genital region. Liver involvement with HSV occurs in neonates, pregnant women, and immunocompromised patients [18]. There are three categories of neonatal HSV infections: local (skin, eye, and mouth) disease, encephalitis, and disseminated infection (with hepatitis) [19]. There is significant neonatal mortality with disseminated disease (60%), and a neonatal mortality rate of 15% with encephalitis. Complications of neonatal HSV infection also include disseminated intravascular coagulopathy and hemorrhagic pneumonitis [20]. Neonatal herpes infection is associated with long-term morbidity; only 40% of survivors are normal following encephalitis or disseminated disease.

Factors that predict neonatal HSV transmission include cervical HSV shedding, invasive fetal monitoring (scalp monitors), preterm delivery, maternal age less than 21 years, and maternal HSV viral load [11]. The majority of neonatal infections can be attributed to maternal genital lesions. Prolonged rupture of membranes may increase the likelihood of transmission. In such cases, cesarean delivery may reduce the risk. Infants may also become infected by contact with the hands of an adult with a non-genital infection.

HSV hepatitis is a difficult diagnosis to establish, and the infection is often fatal. An infant with neonatal herpes infection may be systemically ill. The infant may have hepatosplenomegaly, jaundice, coagulopathy, cutaneous lesions, encephalitis, and seizures [21, 22]. If there is HSV-associated fulminant hepatitis, the prognosis is poor despite antiviral therapy and potential for liver transplantation [7, 10, 21].

Herpes liver disease is characterized by necrosis of hepatocytes and giant cell transformation [23]. Herpes intranuclear inclusion bodies may be found in hepatocytes (Fig. 4). These inclusions are smaller than those of CMV and usually do not appear in bile ducts. Herpes simplex viral DNA may be detected by PCR of blood (Table 1). This test is widely available and may be done rapidly, so it has essentially replaced serologic testing in clinical practice. In cases where there are typical vesicular skin lesions which may be tested, a scraping of an ulcer base may be tested for herpes by direct fluorescent antibody staining, cell culture, or enzyme immunoassay detection of herpes antigens. Liver culture or immunohistochemical staining of liver tissue can also demonstrate the presence of herpes [24].

Herpes infection of the newborn is lethal without treatment [7]. Acyclovir has been the recommended therapy due to its low toxicity. Treatment with acyclovir has been successful in infants with severe liver disease, allowing recovery or creating an opportunity for a life-saving liver transplant [8].

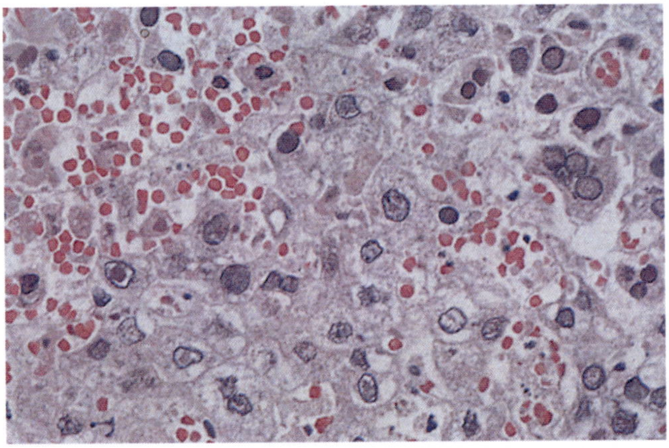

Fig. 4 Pathological findings in herpes simplex hepatitis. Hepatocyte necrosis, multinucleated hepatocytes and many nuclei with eosinophillic viral (Cowdry type A) inclusions. (From *Lucas SB: Other viral and infectious diseases and HIV-related liver disease. In MacSween RNM, Burt AD, Portmann BC, et al [eds]: Pathology of the Liver, 4th ed. London, Churchill Livingstone, 2001, p. 366*)

Human Herpesvirus 6

Serologic studies indicate that human herpesvirus 6 (HHV-6) infects 90% of children by 2 years of age [25, 26]. The peak age of acquisition is between 9 and 21 months. The acquisition of HHV-6 is associated with having older siblings.

Children with primary HHV-6 infection are likely to be symptomatic and have fever, fussiness, diarrhea, rash, and roseola, and are likely to seek medical evaluation. Roseola occurs in a minority of patients, and febrile seizures are infrequently associated with primary HHV-6 infection. Syncytial giant cell hepatitis as well as acute-onset liver failure with HHV-6 infection has been described in children [25, 26]. Testing may be done by PCR assays on tissue or blood (Table 1). Primary infection is usually self-limited and does not require treatment. However, in immunocompromised patients (i.e., liver transplant recipient), active infection or reactivation of HHV-6 can result in rash, myelosuppression, hepatitis, pneumonitis and neurologic disease. In these cases, treatment of established HHV-6 disease is usually intravenous ganciclovir, cidofovir, or foscarnet along with reduced immunosuppression [27].

Non-Herpes Family Viruses

Rubella Virus

Rubella virus (RV) is a member of the family Togaviridiae and the sole member of the genus, Rubivirus. RV contains RNA, which is surrounded by a capsid and a lipoprotein envelope. The capsid and envelope proteins induce the major immune responses.

Rubella is strictly a human disease [1]. Before the introduction of vaccination programs, rubella was endemic worldwide and epidemics occurred every 4–7 years. Rubella vaccines are usually combined with measles and mumps vaccines. Their use has enabled some industrialized countries such as the USA and Scandinavian countries to eliminate rubella and congenital rubella [2]. Rubella is transmitted by aerosol via the respiratory tract. Contact with nasopharyngeal secretions or urine may cause new infections [1].

Congenital rubella was discussed previously. Rubella is generally a mild disease in children, but may be more severe in adults. Depending on the population, 20–50% of infections are subclinical. Rubella has a characteristic nonconfluent maculopapular rash, which appears first on the face and spreads rapidly to the trunk and limbs; lymphadenopathy (suboccipital, postauricular, and cervical lymph nodes) and headache, sore throat, cough, and conjunctivitis may also occur. Arthralgia and arthritis, lasting 4 days to 4 weeks, occur in up to 70% of postpubertal females, but are relatively uncommon in prepubertal children and males. Another serious complication is post-infectious encephalopathy (about 1 in 6,000 cases). Hepatic involvement in congenital rubella usually manifests as hepatomegaly, splenomegaly, jaundice, and cholestasis. Liver histology is nonspecific with giant cell transformation, mononuclear inflammatory infiltrates in portal zones with extramedullary hematopoeisis. There is often cholestasis and bile duct proliferation with varying degrees of intralobular fibrosis [5, 28]. Rubella and congenital rubella are usually diagnosed by detection of rubella-specific IgM; it may be difficult to confirm a diagnosis of congenital rubella in children over 3 months of age [1]. Outside of the newborn period, rubella hepatitis is rare. The more common clinical manifestations of rubella in older children or adults include arthropathy, acute encephalitis, and thrombocytopenia.

Enterovirus

Enteroviruses are small (30 nm), nonenveloped, single-stranded RNA viruses that belong to the family Picornaviridae. There are more than 70 serotypes and they are ubiquitous pathogens worldwide. The 70 known serotypes of enterovirus include echovirus (31 serotypes), coxsackievirus A [23], coxscakievirus B [6], enterovirus 68–71 [4], and poliovirus [3]. Enteroviruses cause more than 15–20 million infections in the USA. Epidemics of enterovirus occur predominantly in the summer and fall. Young children are most likely to be affected, particularly 1–4 years old. In addition to young age, low socioeconomic status and crowding are risk factors for developing enteroviral infections. Since polio has been mostly eliminated from the world via vaccination, the non-polio enteroviruses (NPEV) are the focus of this discussion. NPEV infections account for 30% of reported viral illnesses. Most infections are benign but are capable of causing catastrophic infections in the early newborn period and in very young children during epidemics.

Transmission is mainly fecal–oral and less commonly by respiratory droplets. The virus enters through oral or respiratory mucosa and then replicates in the lymphoid tissue before spreading systemically to cause viremia. Once it is circulating, enterovirus may seed the nervous system, heart, liver, and lungs.

NPEV infections are common, with the majority being, minor, nonspecific febrile illnesses that resolve quickly. In such cases, symptoms include fever, malaise, vomiting, diarrhea, respiratory symptoms, and rash. In addition to nonspecific illness, enteroviral infections cause distinct syndromes such as hand–foot–mouth disease, herpangina, and hemorrhagic conjunctivitis. The clinical disease with NPEV infections may range from minor respiratory illness to aseptic meningitis, encephalitis, acute hemorrhagic conjunctivitis, myocarditis, paralysis, and multiple organ dysfunction syndrome. NPEV infections account for 80–92% of all identifiable causes of aseptic meningitis. NPEV infection may also lead to myocarditis with the development of chronic disease such as dilated cardiomyopathy and congestive heart failure.

In infants, these viral infections are usually self-limited and in several cases of childhood hepatitis due to enterovirus, there was slow but complete resolution of the disease [29]. However, there are reports of jaundice, hepatitis, and progressive hepatic failure with death in neonates with enteroviral infections [26, 30].Echovirus 11 is particularly virulent, causing hepatocellular necrosis and meningoencephalitis that is often fatal. Coxsackie B viruses can produce neonatal myocardial injury [31].

PCR can rapidly and accurately detect enterovirus in urine, serum, CSF, or throat swabs. Serology is a slow diagnostic test that does not distinguish between serotypes, and viral culture is half as sensitive as PCR and slow to grow. Effective antiviral drugs for enterovirus infections are neither licensed nor currently available, although an experimental drug called Pleconaril has shown great efficacy and safety in treatment of enterovirus (Table 1). Pleconaril is an antiviral drug that prevents viral uncoating and attachment to host cell receptors. It has shown efficacy in the treatment of enteroviral meningitis and in immunocompromised patients with severe infection, with 75% of patients having improvement in their symptoms. It has also been used in the treatment of neonatal echovirus and Coxsackie B infections with severe hepatitis.

Parvovirus

Parvovirus is a single-stranded DNA virus transmitted through human blood and respiratory secretions. In most individuals, infection is associated with a self-limited illness characterized by fever, myalgia, and mild myelosuppression. In susceptible hosts, parvovirus may cause more severe or chronic disease such as aplastic crisis in children with hemoglobinopathies, chronic myelosuppression in children with congenital or acquired immunodeficiencies, and hydrops fetalis with fetal demise. Severe interstitial pneumonitis and cholestatic hepatitis have been reported. Laboratory diagnosis can be made by testing for parvovirus B19 IgM antibody although, PCR testing is also available (Table 1).

Parvovirus has been associated with mild acute hepatitis, prolonged severe cholestatic hepatitis, and even acute liver failure in children [19]. In reported cases of severe cholestatic hepatitis, the cholestasis and aminotransferase elevations lasted up to

9 months and appeared to improve with intravenous immunoglobulin therapy. Liver biopsy revealed microvesicular steatosis and cholestasis [32]. Treatment is generally not warranted unless there is severe hepatitis or aplastic anemia or immunocompromise at which point use of intravenous immunoglobulin would be considered.

Reovirus

The family Reoviridae (*r*espiratory *e*nteric *o*rphan viruses) includes four viruses causing human disease: orthoreovirus, orbivirus, coltivirus, and rotavirus. The reoviruses commonly infect humans but infrequently cause human disease. Upper respiratory infections, exanthems, pneumonia, hepatitis, encephalitis, gastroenteritis, and biliary atresia have on occasion been associated with these viruses.

Reovirus 3 has been proposed as a candidate for the etiologic agent of biliary atresia and neonatal hepatitis based on the presence of antibodies in the sera of affected infants and the pattern of infection in the livers of weanling mice. However, there has been no confirmation of this association to date [12].

Paramyxovirus

Paramyxoviridae are nonsegmented, negative-sense, single-stranded RNA viruses (Fig. 3d). This family is divided into the *Paramyxoviridae* subfamily containing *Respirovirus* (Sendai virus, parainfluenza virus type 3), *Rubulavirus* (mumps, parainfluenza virus type 2), and *Morbillivirus* (measles) genera; and *Pneumoviridae* subfamily (*Pneumovirus* genus [respiratory syncytial virus]).

A nonspecific clinical illness with diarrhea and then the development of jaundice and liver failure has been reported in a previously well 6-week-old male infant with paramyxovirus [26]. Giant cell hepatitis with a significant mixed lymphocytic and neutrophilic infiltrate was present on both wedge and core biopsies. The residual 60% of hepatocytes had ballooning degeneration and many possessed pyknotic nuclei. The hepatocytes were arranged in a pseudoacinar pattern. Electron microscopy showed paramyxovirus-like inclusions in the giant cells, characterized as large inclusions with fine filamentous, beaded substructures (18–20 nm) [26]. In this case, as in most viral hepatitis, supportive care is given and if there is nonresolving fulminant liver failure, then liver transplantation is offered [26] (Table 1).

HIV

The World Health Organization estimated that more than 33 million persons worldwide were living with HIV infection at the end of 2009, 60% of these are women and children under 15 years of age [33]. The primary route of infection in the pediatric population is vertical transmission. The other common routes of transmission include sexual contact with an infected individual and exposure to infected blood or blood products. Maternal zidovudine (ZDV) treatment during pregnancy and labor, and neonatal ZDV therapy for the first 6 weeks of life reduced the relative risk of vertical transmission of HIV by 66%. Mothers and infants who did not receive ZDV had a 25.5% chance of vertical transmission, compared to 8.3% in those who received the antiretroviral drug. Combination regimens with ZDV plus a second antiretroviral agent such as lamivudine have shown even greater efficacy at prevention of HIV transmission. The combination of ZDV chemoprophylaxis with additional antiretroviral drugs for treatment of HIV infection is recommended for infected women whose clinical, immunologic, or virologic status requires treatment and should be strongly considered for any infected woman with an HIV RNA rate > 1,000 copies/mL, regardless of clinical or immunologic status, and can be considered for women with HIV RNA rate < 1,000 copies/mL [34]. Other infections such as hepatitis B and C may be transmitted more efficiently when the mother is coinfected with HIV. Vertical transmission of HCV is 3.8 times higher in HIV coinfected women. Since the early 1990s, the annual number of diagnoses of perinatally acquired AIDS and HIV infection has declined by approximately 90% in the USA as a result of routine HIV screening of pregnant women and the availability of effective interventions to prevent transmission [33].

Most infants with vertically-acquired HIV infection have a normal physical examination at birth, and then start to develop subtle signs and symptoms which may include lymphadenopathy, hepatosplenomegaly, failure to thrive, chronic or recurrent diarrhea, interstitial pneumonia, and oral thrush. Some of the clinical manifestations seen more commonly in children than in adults are recurrent bacterial infections, chronic parotid swelling, lymphocytic interstitial pneumonitis, and early onset of progressive neurologic deterioration. Opportunistic infections are seen with severe depression of CD4 counts.

The most common opportunistic infections are *Pneumocystis carinii* pneumonia (PCP) and *Mycobacterium avium* complex (MAC). Fungal infections can include oral candidiasis, Candida esophagitis, rarely disseminated histoplasmosis, and coccidioidomycosis or cryptococcocis. Parasitic infections include intestinal crytosporidiosis, microsporidiosis, giardiasis, or isosporiasis. Viral infections include recurrent or persistent HSV, VZV, CMV, or measles [35].

Although severe hepatic dysfunction is not a common manifestation of HIV disease in pediatrics, more than 90% of HIV-infected children have hepatosplenomegaly at some time during the course of infection. In HIV disease, chronic liver inflammation with or without cholestasis is often present without an identified etiology. Some of the identified pathogens in HIV-related liver disease include cryptosporidial cholecystitis, and chronic hepatitis with CMV, HBV, HCV, or MAC. These may lead to cirrhosis and liver failure [35, 36]. Granulomatous disease of the liver is most commonly due to mycobacterial or fungal agents, but sometimes found in the absence of identifiable infection (Fig. 5) (Table 1). Several antiretroviral drugs such as protease inhibitors, didanosine, and dapsone cause reversible aminotransferase elevations. While liver

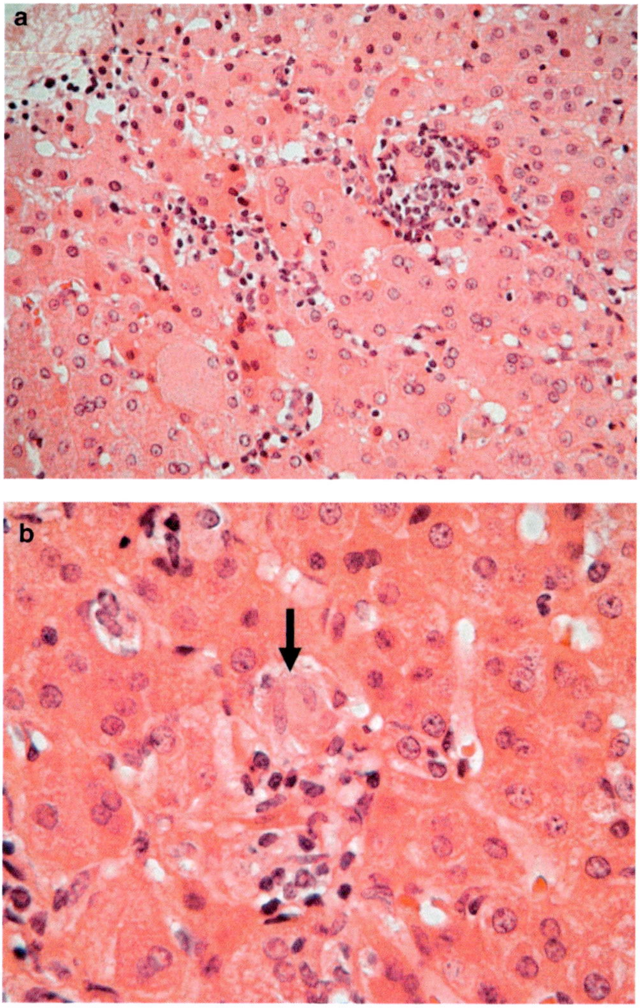

Fig. 5 Pathological findinds in HIV disease. Biopsy from 1 year old with HIV and elevated transaminases. Histology shows: (**a**) extensive portal and lobular inflammation of chronic inflammatory cells, (**b**) tiny collections of epitheliod histiocytes–granulomatous hepatitis

disease may progress more rapidly in adults coinfected with HCV and HIV, it is not known if this is the case in children. Transplantation in HIV-infected patients is at the forefront of clinical medicine, challenging medical therapy and stimulating ethical discussions. Recent data from HIV-infected adults receiving OLT suggest that liver transplantation can be successful in properly selected HIV-infected patients who are receiving recommended treatment.

In summary, the non A–E viral infections tend to affect the liver as one component of a systemic infection which involves other organ systems. The severity of the liver disease seen with these infections is predicated by the maturity and competence of the hosts' immune system. Neonates and immunocompromised individuals may develop a life-threatening disease that warrants antiviral therapy, whereas an immunocompetent host would be more likely to have a self-limited illness. Awareness of these differences should help direct therapy of these infections.

References

1. Best JM. Rubella. Semin Fetal Neonatal Med 2007;12(3):182–92.
2. Muller CP, Kremer JR, Best JM, Dourado I, Triki H, Reef S. Reducing global disease burden of measles and rubella: report of the WHO Steering Committee on research related to measles and rubella vaccines and vaccination, 2005. Vaccine 2007;25(1):1–9.
3. Lanari M, Lazzarotto T, Venturi V, et al. Neonatal cytomegalovirus blood load and risk of sequelae in symptomatic and asymptomatic congenitally infected newborns. Pediatrics 2006;117(1):e76–83.
4. Yamamoto AY, Mussi-Pinhata MM, Cristina P, Pinto G, Moraes Figueiredo LT, Jorge SM. Congenital cytomegalovirus infection in preterm and full-term newborn infants from a population with a high seroprevalence rate. Pediatr Infect Dis J 2001;20(2):188–92.
5. Watkins JB, Sunaryo FP, Berezin SH. Hepatic manifestations of congenital and perinatal disease. Clin Perinatol 1981;8(3):467–80.
6. Munro SC, Trincado D, Hall B, Rawlinson WD. Symptomatic infant characteristics of congenital cytomegalovirus disease in Australia. J Paediatr Child Health 2005;41(8):449–52.
7. Meerbach A, Sauerbrei A, Meerbach W, Bittrich HJ, Wutzler P. Fatal outcome of herpes simplex virus type 1-induced necrotic hepatitis in a neonate. Med Microbiol Immunol 2006; 195(2):101–5.
8. Egawa H, Inomata Y, Nakayama S, et al. Fulminant hepatic failure secondary to herpes simplex virus infection in a neonate: a case report of successful treatment with liver transplantation and perioperative acyclovir. Liver Transpl Surg 1998;4(6):513–5.
9. D'Andrea CC, Ferrera PC. Disseminated herpes simplex virus infection in a neonate. Am J Emerg Med 1998;16(4):376–8.
10. Jain R, Shareef M, Rowley A, Raible MD, Husain AN, Myers TF. Disseminated herpes simplex virus infection presenting as fever in the newborn – a lethal outcome. J Infect 1996;32(3):239–41.
11. Fortran S. Systemic Viral Infections that may Involve the Liver. In: Fortram S (ed) Feldman: Sleisenger & Fordtran's Gastrointestinal and Liver Disease, 8th ed. Saunders, Philadelphia; 2006.
12. Rosenthal P. Neonatal Hepatitis and Congenital Infections. In: Suchy F (ed.), Liver Disease in Children, Mosby, St. Louis, Missouri 2008;235–41.
13. Ozkan TB, Mistik R, Dikici B, Nazlioglu HO. Antiviral therapy in neonatal cholestatic cytomegalovirus hepatitis. BMC Gastroenterol 2007;7:9.
14. Zuppan CW, Bui HD, Grill BG. Diffuse hepatic fibrosis in congenital cytomegalovirus infection. J Pediatr Gastroenterol Nutr 1986;5(3):489–91.
15. Dresler S, Linder D. Noncirrhotic portal fibrosis following neonatal cytomegalic inclusion disease. J Pediatr 1978;93(5):887–8.
16. Cohen JI. Epstein-Barr Virus Infection. N Engl J Med 2000;343(7):481–92.
17. Mendez-Sanchez N, Aguilar-Dominguez C, Chavez-Tapia NC, Uribe M. Hepatic manifestations of Epstein-Barr viral infection. Ann Hepatol 2005;4(3):205–9.
18. Kaufman B, Gandhi SA, Louie E, Rizzi R, Illei P. Herpes simplex virus hepatitis: case report and review. Clin Infect Dis 1997;24(3):334–8.

19. Aydin M, Bulut Y, Poyrazoglu G, Turgut M, Seyrek A. Detection of human parvovirus B19 in children with acute hepatitis. Ann Trop Paediatr 2006;26(1):25–8.
20. Kesson AM. Management of neonatal herpes simplex virus infection. Paediatr Drugs 2001; 3(2):81–90.
21. Benador N, Mannhardt W, Schranz D, et al. Three cases of neonatal herpes simplex virus infection presenting as fulminant hepatitis. Eur J Pediatr 1990;149(8):555–9.
22. Philippe I, Anne Marie Roque A, Mylène S, et al. Herpes simplex virus-associated acute liver failure: a difficult diagnosis with a poor prognosis. Liver Transpl 2005;11(12):1550–5.
23. Singer DB. Pathology of neonatal Herpes simplex virus infection. Perspect Pediatr Pathol 1981;6:243–78.
24. Nakamura Y, Yamamoto S, Tanaka S, et al. Herpes simplex viral infection in human neonates: an immunohistochemical and electron microscopic study. Hum Pathol 1985;16(11):1091–7.
25. Zerr DM, Meier AS, Selke SS, et al. A population-based study of primary human herpesvirus 6 infection. N Engl J Med 2005;352(8):768–76.
26. Hicks J, Barrish J, Zhu SH. Neonatal syncytial giant cell hepatitis with paramyxoviral-like inclusions. Ultrastruct Pathol 2001;25(1):65–71.
27. Abdel RC, Razonable RR. Human herpesvirus 6 infections after liver transplantation. World J Gastroenterol 2009;15(21):2561–9
28. Strauss L, Bernstein J. Neonatal hepatitis in congenital rubella. A histopathological study. Arch Pathol 1968;86(3):317–27.
29. Kawashima H, Ryou S, Nishimata S, et al. Enteroviral hepatitis in children. Pediatr Int 2004;46(2):130–4.
30. Pino-Ramirez RM, Pertierra-Cortada A, Iriondo-Sanz M, Krauel-Vidal X, Munoz-Almagro C. Neonatal echovirus 30 infection associated with severe hepatitis in twin neonates. Pediatr Infect Dis J 2008;27(1):88.
31. Nathan M, Walsh R, Hardin JT, et al. Enteroviral sepsis and ischemic cardiomyopathy in a neonate: case report and review of literature. Asaio J 2008;54(5):554–5.
32. Bousvaros A, Sundel R, Thorne GM, et al. Parvovirus B19-associated interstitial lung disease, hepatitis, and myositis. Pediatr Pulmonol 1998;26(5):365–9.
33. CDC. Global AIDS Report. 2010.
34. Dao H, Mofenson LM, Ekpini R, et al. International recommendations on antiretroviral drugs for treatment of HIV-infected women and prevention of mother-to-child HIV transmission in resource-limited settings: 2006 update. Am J Obstet Gynecol 2007;197(3 Suppl):S42–55.
35. Poles MA, Dieterich DT, Schwarz ED, et al. Liver biopsy findings in 501 patients infected with human immunodeficiency virus (HIV). J Acquir Immune Defic Syndr Hum Retrovirol 1996;11(2):170–7.
36. Schneiderman DJ, Arenson DM, Cello JP, Margaretten W, Weber TE. Hepatic disease in patients with the acquired immune deficiency syndrome (AIDS). Hepatology 1987;7(5): 925–30.

Immunoprophylaxis of Hepatitis A and Hepatitis B in Children

Scott A. Elisofon

Key Concepts

- Hepatitis A vaccines are extremely safe, immunogenic, and effective in prevention of infection. Universal childhood vaccination is recommended.
- Since implementation of newer hepatitis A vaccination strategies in 1995, the incidence of infection has decreased by over 92%.
- Hepatitis A vaccine may now be used as postexposure prophylaxis for most children over the age of 1 year.
- The incidence of acute hepatitis B has decreased by 98% since 1990, mostly due to improved vaccination strategies.
- Hepatitis B vaccine and hepatitis B immune globulin must be given promptly to infants born to hepatitis B-infected mothers and unvaccinated persons with hepatitis B exposure.

Keywords Hepatitis A vaccine • Immune globulin • Hepatitis B vaccine • Hepatitis B immune globulin

Introduction

Although hepatitis A virus (HAV) and hepatitis B virus (HBV) are different in terms of virology and transmission, both of these infections are almost completely preventable with proper immunoprophylaxis, implemented either prior to or after exposure to infection. Vaccines for both have been available for many years: the first effective HBV vaccine was released almost 40 years ago, and HAV vaccines

S.A. Elisofon (✉)
Division of Gastroenterology and Nutrition, Children's Hospital Boston,
300 Longwood Avenue, Boston, MA 02115, USA
e-mail: scott.elisofon@childrens.harvard.edu

M.M. Jonas (ed.), *Viral Hepatitis in Children: Unique Features and Opportunities*,
Clinical Gastroenterology, DOI 10.1007/978-1-60761-373-2_8,

were licensed in the early 1990s. With widespread use over the last 15 years, remarkable drops in the rates of acute infections have been observed [1]. This chapter will describe the available vaccines and immunoglobulins used for pre- and postexposure prophylaxis, and discuss indications, short- and long-term efficacy data, and safety.

Hepatitis A

Hepatitis A is an RNA virus that spreads via the fecal-oral route, and occasionally via shared needles from someone actively viremic [2–4]. Young children can present with acute gastroenteritis symptoms without evidence of hepatitis or jaundice. They may actively shed virus for weeks to months and serve as an important source of infection in the community. To prevent individual cases as well as outbreaks, active immunization and occasionally passive immunization are required, and the recommendations will be discussed below.

Passive Immunization: Immune Globulin

Immune globulin (IG) is a preparation of pooled human plasma processed by cold ethanol fractionation [5]. In the USA, this plasma must be screened for infections, including hepatitis B, hepatitis C, and human immunodeficiency virus (HIV) prior to use, and the US Food and Drug Administration (FDA) mandates that there be a viral inactivation step or that the final IG tests HCV RNA negative by polymerase chain reaction (PCR) [6]. HAV concentrations vary among lots, and there are reports of lower concentrations in more recent preparations, as fewer donors have been infected. Despite these concerns, there is no documentation of decreased efficacy of IG in the prevention of HAV infection [6].

IG can be used in children younger than 12 months of age for both pre- and postexposure prophylaxes. It is given intramuscularly (IM) and transfers HAV antibody to the recipient. Dosing is 0.02 mL/kg for pre- or postexposure prophylaxis. It can be given as prophylaxis in a single dose for short periods of exposure (under 3 months) or repeated doses for exposures of greater than 5 months. Efficacy of this product was first reported in 1945, and it has been in continuous use since then [7]. Preexposure prophylaxis efficacy is excellent, and postexposure efficacy has been demonstrated to be 80–90% [2, 6]. IG is available in single-dose or multi-dose vials.

IG is considered a very safe product, and serious adverse events are uncommon, but anaphylactic reactions have been described. In particular, there are reports of anaphylactic reactions from repetitive IG dosages in IgA-deficient individuals. IG is therefore contraindicated in this population [6, 8]. However, there are no specific recommendations for checking IgA levels prior to single or repeated doses.

IG may prevent an immune response from several live, attenuated vaccines such as measles, mumps, and rubella (MMR) and varicella if they are provided concurrently [9, 10]. Further consultation with an infectious disease specialist may be warranted if IG is to be given at or around the time of administration of these vaccines.

Active Immunization: Vaccine

Formalin-inactivated HAV vaccines were developed in the early 1990s and approved for use in 1995 after several trials in children demonstrated immunogenicity and safety [11, 12]. Vaccine production includes a virus inactivation step similar to that used for the inactivated poliovirus vaccine [13, 14]. Once inactivated, the HAV is bound to an aluminum hydroxide adjuvant.

Currently, there are two HAV vaccines approved by the FDA for both children and adults: Havrix® (GlaxoSmithKline, Rixensart, Belgium) and Vaqta® (Merck & Co., Inc., Whitehouse Station, NJ). A combination HAV/HBV vaccine is approved for persons 18 years and older (Twinrix®, GlaxoSmithKline). HAV vaccine doses are expressed in the quantity of HAV antigen per vaccination; Havrix® and Twinrix® use enzyme-linked immunoassay units (EL.U) and Vaqta® units (U).

Vaccine should be given intramuscularly, and primary doses are followed with secondary vaccination 6–18 months later for Havrix® and Vaqta®. One study has demonstrated interchangeability of these preparations in sequential dosing of the same individuals [15]. Twinrix® is provided in the schedule recommended for the hepatitis B series (Table 1).

Immunogenicity

Several studies have shown superb immunogenicity and efficacy in prevention of hepatitis A in healthy children who received HAV vaccination [16–19]. Two large,

Table 1 Hepatitis A and B vaccines

Vaccine	Age	Dose	Schedule
Hepatitis A			
Havrix®[a]	12 months–18 years	720 EL.U	0, 6–12 months
Vaqta®[b]	12 months–18 years	25 U	0, 6–12 months
Hepatitis B			
Recombivax-HB[b]	0–19 years	5 μg	0, 1, 6 months
Engerix-B[a]	0–19 years	10 μg	0, 1, 6 months
Hepatitis A and B			
Twinrix®[a]	≥18 years	720 EL.U (HAV) 20 μg (HBV)	0, 1, 6 months

EL.U enzyme-linked immunoassay units, *U* units
[a]GlaxoSmithKline Biologicals, Rixensart, Belgium
[b]Merck & Co., Inc., Whitehouse Station, NJ

randomized, placebo-controlled trials in children aged 1–16 years, conducted in New York (1,000 patients) and Thailand (40,000 patients), demonstrated protection from HAV infection in 94–100% of children who received two doses of vaccine [11, 12].

Several studies have documented decreased HAV vaccine immunogenicity in infants born to mothers who are seropositive for antibody to HAV (anti-HAV) [20, 21]. However, although total antibody concentrations are lower in this population, the majority are still protected from infection. Given that the majority of passively acquired HAV antibody disappears by age 1, vaccination beginning at this age appears to be successful [22, 23].

Immunocompromised individuals tolerate HAV vaccination well, with good safety profiles. However, there are some conflicting data as to HAV vaccination success in this mixed population. In one small study of 32 immunized HIV-infected children with higher CD4 counts (>300 cells/mm^3), 100% developed protective antibody levels [24]. However, other studies have demonstrated less success, especially in children with lower CD4 counts [25, 26].

Studies of liver transplant recipients demonstrate lower immunogenicity of HAV vaccine than that in the normal population [27]. This has been demonstrated in both adult and pediatric cohorts [27, 28]. In addition, there are reports of waning immunity in adults who received liver or kidney transplants [29]. The authors suggest that boosters should be considered, but there are no official recommendations for this population. Currently, there are no data on the use of HAV vaccine in stem cell transplant recipients, and hence there are no specific recommendations for this population [30, 31]. There have been suggestions that the vaccine could be considered in stem cell recipients who have liver disease from chronic graft-versus-host disease (GVHD) or other viruses, in addition to those living in communities where HAV is endemic [30].

Early reports of immunogenicity in adults with chronic liver disease demonstrated safety but fewer seroconversions than that in healthy populations [32]. However, three recent studies conducted in children showed good immunogenicity and safety profiles [33–35]. Although these studies were small, they documented 97–100% seroconversion one month after the second HAV vaccination. Vaccination is recommended for all children greater than 1 year of age with chronic liver disease, including those listed for liver transplant.

Long-Term Immunogenicity

Long-term immunogenicity and efficacy have been evaluated in several studies in children up to 10 years after vaccination [36, 37]. A 6-year follow-up of 549 children who received Vaqta® showed that 544 (99%) had protective levels of HAV antibody [38]. Recently, 100% of a cohort of Alaskan children was found to have HAV antibody 10 years after vaccination [36].

Long-term efficacy in HAV prevention has been demonstrated in the New York cohort from the Vaqta® trial, with 9-year follow-up documenting no cases of HAV infection in the immunized children [37]. Further studies are necessary for longer term immunity and efficacy assessment.

Adverse Reactions

Both licensed HAV vaccines are extremely safe. In clinical studies of both Havrix® and Vaqta®, the most common complaints in children included pain, tenderness or warmth at injection sites (18–39%), feeding problems, or headache (less than 15%) [11, 12]. Serious adverse events have not been identified in association with HAV vaccines [6].

Preexposure Prophylaxis (Table 2)

Children <1 Year of Age

For infants less than 1 year of age, IG is the only approved prophylaxis, recommended for travel to medium- or high-endemic regions (see Fig. 1). Intramuscular IG at 0.02 mL/kg will confer protection from HAV infection for 3 months. For trips that are longer than 3 months, larger doses can be given (0.06 mL/kg), for protection up to 5 months. Repeat doses can be given every 5 months if the infant remains in the area of high prevalence [6].

Children ≥1 Year of Age

Since 1995, vaccines have been approved by the FDA for children aged 2 years and older. In 1996, the Advisory Committee on Immunization Practices (ACIP) of the Centers for Disease Control (CDC) suggested vaccination for persons at increased risk of infection or persons interested in obtaining immunity. It was further suggested that routine immunization be performed in children above 2 years of age

Table 2 Immunoprophylaxis summary for Hepatitis A [6, 41]

Preexposure prophylaxis	
<1 year	IG (0.02 mL/kg)
1–18 years	Hepatitis A vaccine series
Immunocompromised	Hepatitis A vaccine and consider IG[a]
Chronic liver disease	Hepatitis A vaccine and consider IG[a]
Postexposure prophylaxis (within 2 weeks)	
Previously immunized	No intervention
<1 year	IG
1–18 years (healthy)	Hepatitis A vaccine series
Immunocompromised	IG and consider vaccine[b]
Chronic liver disease	IG and consider vaccine[b]

IG immune globulin
[a]IG should be given if a person is traveling to a region of high endemicity, and if there is concern for decreased immune response to the vaccine
[b]IG is recommended, but vaccine should be considered in addition

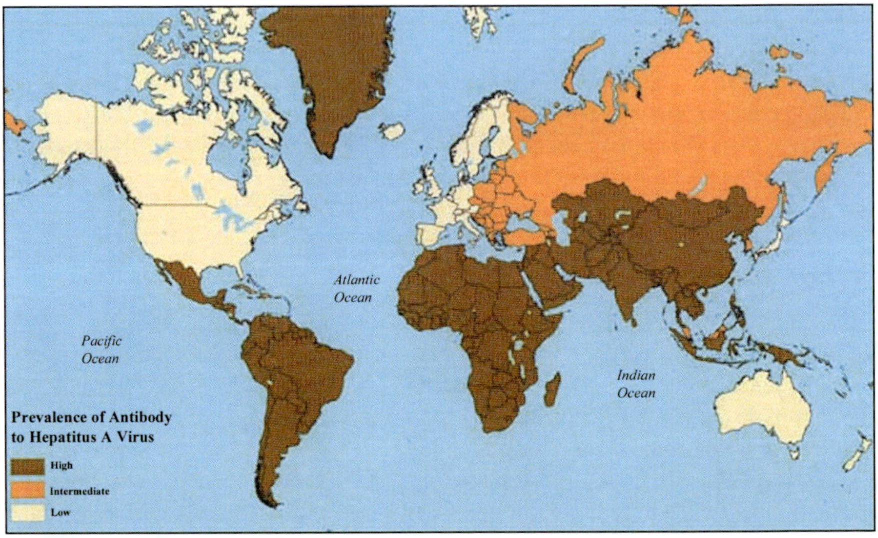

Fig. 1 Prevalence of antibody to hepatitis A virus (from www.cdc.gov) [130]

who lived in high-prevalence regions of the USA, as well as in those with chronic liver disease and those traveling to HAV-endemic countries.

In 1999, the ACIP recommended routine vaccination of all children living in areas of the USA that had HAV incidence rates of at least 20 per 100,000 (Alaska, Arizona, California, Idaho, Nevada, New Mexico, Oklahoma, Oregon, South Dakota, Utah, and Washington) and consideration of vaccination in states (Arkansas, Colorado, Missouri, Montana, Texas, and Wyoming) and counties with more than 10 per 100,000 during that time period [39]. These recommendations for vaccination were reviewed 4 years later, in 2003, and an 88% decline of acute HAV infection in those states with suggested routine vaccination was documented [40].

In 2005, HAV vaccine was recommended for children down to 12 months of age, which enabled this immunization to be incorporated into routine childhood vaccination programs.

In 2006, new recommendations were published from the ACIP regarding preexposure prophylaxis, to further reduce HAV incidence and morbidity [6]. These recommendations for children include the following (Table 2):

- Vaccination for all children 12–23 months of age. Children not vaccinated by age 2 years should be vaccinated in subsequent visits.
- States, counties, and communities with existing HAV vaccine programs for children aged 2–18 years should maintain them.
- In areas without existing HAV vaccine programs, catch-up vaccination of unvaccinated children aged 2–18 years should be considered.

The most recent data from 2007 show a 92% decline in the incidence of HAV infection from 12 cases per 100,000 in 1995 to 1 case per 100,000 population in 2007 [1].

Groups At High Risk

In addition to recommendations for universal childhood HAV vaccination, the ACIP has recommended preexposure prophylaxis for people at increased risk of infection, and has made further updates on international travel and adoption (Table 3) [6, 41, 42].

If children aged 12 months or older are known to be traveling to HAV-endemic areas, vaccination is recommended at least 4 weeks in advance, although any time prior to departure can provide adequate protection for healthy people [41]. A second dose should be provided within 6–12 months of the first vaccination. Children less than 1 year of age should be given IG, as stated above. If a child has travel scheduled within 2 weeks, is immunocompromised, or has another chronic medical problem, IG is suggested in addition to vaccine [6, 41].

Within the last year, the ACIP has instituted a recommendation that all unvaccinated persons who will have close, personal contact with an international adoptee from a medium- or high-endemic region within the first 60 days following arrival in the USA receive HAV vaccine [42].

Data have shown that the vaccination rate in men who have sex with men appears to be low [43]. All adolescents in this group should be immunized.

In the USA, there have been increasing reports of HAV outbreaks in persons using injection and noninjection illicit drugs, such as methamphetamine [3, 4]. This mode of drug abuse has accounted for almost half of the outbreaks of HAV infection in this population. All users of injection and noninjection illicit drugs should be vaccinated for HAV.

The only occupational risk recognized at this time is working with nonhuman primates [44]. Vaccination of food handlers or employees in waste management (sewerage) systems is not routinely recommended [6].

Children who receive infusions of clotting-factor concentrates have been more susceptible to parenterally transmitted HAV infection, but this risk is decreasing with more routine vaccination of blood donors [45]. Still, vaccine is recommended at this time for all of these individuals [6].

All patients with chronic liver disease should be vaccinated against HAV [6]. This should include patients who are being listed for or have already received a liver transplant and were not previously immunized.

Table 3 Groups at increased risk for hepatitis A infection

Persons traveling to or working in countries with high or intermediate endemicity
Household contacts of new international adoptees
Men who have sex with men
Users of injection and noninjection illicit drugs
Persons with occupational risk
Individuals with clotting factor disorders
Persons with chronic liver disease

Prevaccination Testing

Prevaccination testing for the presence of anti-HAV is not recommended for most children and adolescents, as their expected prevalence is low and this would not be cost effective [6]. Testing may be considered for older adolescents from endemic populations such as Native Americans, Alaska Natives, and Hispanics.

Postvaccination Testing

Postvaccination testing for seroconversion (i.e., documentation of development of anti-HAV) is not indicated given the high rates of vaccination response outlined above [6].

Postexposure Prophylaxis (Table 2)

Vaccine should be used in all circumstances for postexposure prophylaxis except in infants less than 1 year of age. Exposed persons who have been previously vaccinated for HAV with at least 1 dose, 4 weeks prior to exposure, do not require postexposure prophylaxis. In addition, attendees of elementary and secondary schools, hospitals, or workplaces do not require prophylaxis if the source of infection is not from that setting.

Children who do require prophylaxis include those who are unvaccinated, and fit one of the following criteria:

1. Close personal contact: Household or sexual contacts, babysitters, or persons who share drugs with individuals with documented HAV infection.
2. Child-care centers: Staff members and children, if one or more cases are recognized or two or more households of attendees have reported cases. This is for centers that provide care to children in diapers.
3. Common source exposures: Food handlers who work with an infected food handler should receive prophylaxis. Transmission of infection to patrons is quite unlikely, although recommendations from the CDC suggest consideration of prophylaxis for patrons if the food handler handled uncooked or cooked food and had diarrhea or poor hygiene at the time [6].

Until recently, the postexposure prophylaxis recommendations included IG (0.02 mL/kg) for all unvaccinated persons, within 2 weeks of exposure to HAV infection from close personal contact, child-care centers, or common-source exposures [6]. Data show that this strategy is between 80% and 90% effective in preventing HAV infection [46]. There is no efficacy of IG given more than 2 weeks after exposure.

The promising use of HAV vaccine for postexposure prophylaxis had been reported with recommendations for use in Europe and Canada, initially with no change in recommendations from the ACIP [47, 48]. However, recently, the ACIP has changed its recommendations upon reviewing a randomized, double-blind, noninferiority trial comparing HAV vaccine and IG after exposure to HAV [49]. This study, conducted in Kazakhstan, randomized over 1,000 persons aged 2–40 years who were not already immune to HAV. Most of these were children, and most received treatment after the first week of exposure (mean, 10 days). Symptomatic infection occurred in 4.4% of those who received vaccine versus 3.3% of those who received IG. These data confirmed noninferiority of HAV vaccine as postexposure prophylaxis. Further arguments for the use of HAV vaccine for postexposure prophylaxis include cost equal to IG, long-lasting immunity in vaccine recipients, and prevention of secondary infections from pooled donors for IG [41]. Because of the new data, HAV vaccine is now recommended for postexposure prophylaxis in persons who are unvaccinated to HAV, healthy, and 1–40 years of age. Children who should still receive IG after a known exposure include those under 1 year of age, and those who are immunocompromised, or who have chronic liver disease (Table 2) [41].

Conclusions

Over the past 14 years, the incidence of hepatitis A infection in the USA has drastically decreased, secondary to expanded vaccination strategies, as well as simpler postexposure prophylaxis guidelines. The recommendations for universal immunization for children over 1 year are becoming more accepted throughout the USA, and are easy to incorporate into the standard immunization schedule. This will help to further decrease the incidence of this preventable infection. The vaccine is extremely safe and immunogenic, even in the special populations outlined above. Some high-risk groups are still under-immunized, and efforts to correct this are warranted.

Hepatitis B

Hepatitis B virus (HBV) is a DNA virus, which is transmitted by exposure to blood or bodily fluids through birth, mucosal or percutaneous exposure, or sexual activity. Vertical transmission is the most common cause of chronic infection found in both children and adults. The development of chronic hepatitis B is inversely proportional to the age of acquisition [50]. Since the introduction of the first HBV vaccine in 1982, tremendous progress has been made in reducing the incidence of chronic infection in children. Further progress has been made with expanded immunization practices, which will be discussed.

Passive Immunization: Hepatitis B Immune Globulin

Hepatitis B immune globulin (HBIG) provides antibody to hepatitis B surface antigen (anti-HBs) and passive protection for approximately 3–6 months. It is prepared from the plasma of donors who have high concentrations of anti-HBs.

Like IG, these samples are tested for hepatitis B surface antigen (HBsAg), antibodies to HIV and HCV, and HCV RNA. Each vial or syringe of HBIG is assayed for sufficient anti-HBs titer. Most measurements suggest titers of >220 IU/mL. This is in contrast to IG that does not quantify the titer of anti-HBs.

Indications for HBIG use in pediatrics include perinatal exposure to an HBsAg-positive mother, sexual exposure to an HBsAg-positive person, accidental percutaneous or mucosal exposure to HBV, or receipt of a solid organ transplant from a hepatitis B-infected donor. HBIG is considered a very safe product, with few side effects, comparable to standard IG. HBIG is usually administered in combination with the HBV vaccine [51] (see Postexposure Prophylaxis).

Active Immunization: Hepatitis B Vaccine

Hepatitis B vaccines are prepared with purified fragments of hepatitis B surface proteins, and do not contain intact virus or viral genome. HBsAg was originally purified from the plasma of hepatitis B-infected persons to create the first vaccine, but since 1986, the antigen has been produced by recombinant DNA technology [52]. The surface antigen is obtained from cultures of genetically engineered *Saccharomyces cerevisiae* cells, which carry and express the surface antigen gene of hepatitis B virus. The surface antigen is then purified and formulated as a suspension.

HBV vaccines are available as single-antigen vaccines or in combination with other vaccinations. The two single-antigen vaccines are Recombivax-HB® (Merck & Co., Inc., Whitehouse Station, NJ) and Engerix-B® (GlaxoSmithKline Biologicals, Rixensart, Belgium). Combination vaccines approved for use in children include Comvax® (Merck & Co., Inc.,) which combines HBsAg and *Haemophilus influenzae* type b, and Pediarix® (GlaxoSmithKline) which contains recombinant HBsAg, diphtheria and tetanus toxoids, acellular pertussis adsorbed (DTaP), and inactivated poliovirus. Twinrix® (GlaxoSmithKline), which contains both recombinant HBsAg and inactivated HAV, is approved only for persons aged 18 years and older (Table 1).

The routine schedule for immunization of infants and children against HBV includes three intramuscular injections of the vaccine. Most schedules include doses at birth, 1 month, and 6 months, although other regimens may be used [51]. The dosages recommended and approved for children less than 19 years of age are 5 μg for Recombivax-HB and 10 μg for Engerix-B. These vaccinations appear to be interchangeable for completion of the three-dose series [53]. Combination vaccines are not approved for infants less than 6 weeks, so single-antigen vaccine must be given at birth [51].

Immunogenicity

If administered according to the recommended schedule, the vaccines will induce a protective response in 95% of infants, children, and adolescents [54–57]. An anti-HBs titer of ≥10 mIU/mL is considered the standard cutoff for immunity.

Routine checking of anti-HBs titer is not recommended unless vaccinated children are household contacts of HBV-infected persons [51].

Patients with untreated celiac disease have been shown to have lower seroconversion rates than normal healthy children [58, 59]. This has also been documented in obese patients [60]. A recent publication reported greater success with longer needles, after speculating that increased subcutaneous fat stores may not allow for proper intramuscular dosing of HBV vaccine, leading to an inadequate immune response [61]. Other children who may have difficulty with seroconversion or require additional vaccine doses are described below.

Preterm infants with birth weight under 2,000 g are less likely than full-term infants to develop antibody response to HBV vaccines administered in the first month of life [62–64]. After the first month, antibody responses appear equal to those of term infants [65, 66]. Given these data, the ACIP and AAP recommend waiting for 1 month prior to implementing vaccination in preterm infants born at less than 2,000 g to HBsAg-negative mothers [51]. If the infant is stable and ready for discharge prior to 30 days, immunization should be given. If infants are born to HBsAg-positive women or those with unknown HBsAg status, vaccine should be given at birth, but it is not counted as part of the three-dose series.

There are limited data on pediatric hemodialysis patients and their response to standard HBV vaccination protocols. However, anti-HBs titers should be obtained in these children after completing the series. Several published reports advocate for a higher dose of vaccine and possibly a four-vaccine schedule, with seroconversion rates of 75–97% [67–69].

Seroconversion rates are lower in children with HIV [70–73], those undergoing chemotherapy [74, 75], and those who have received stem cell or solid organ transplants [28, 76, 77]. These patients should have additional boosters, and possibly higher doses may be required if their titers are not sufficient.

Long-Term Immunogenicity

The hepatitis B vaccine series is quite immunogenic, as stated above, with a short-term titer of ≥10mIU/mL induced in close to 95% of healthy children who receive the three-dose series. The long-term duration of antibody and protection against infection in children immunized in infancy and the need for booster doses have been examined. In 2004, Alaskan investigators demonstrated loss of anti-HBs by 5 years in over 60% of infants who had received either plasma-derived or recombinant vaccine [78]. However, most patients did demonstrate immunologic memory with a booster dose and hence were still considered protected. A study from Taiwan demonstrated satisfactory immunity for up to 15 years [79]. Although titers waned after 15 years, they rapidly rebounded after one booster vaccine dose [80]. A group from Hong Kong showed that more than 80% of children immunized with three doses had anti-HBs greater than 10 mIU/ml 12 years later, and that additional booster doses were not required [81]. This cohort was followed for up to 18 years, and continued to demonstrate adequate immunity and effective protection [82]. Despite waning anti-HBs titers, HBsAg carrier rates in endemic populations have dramatically decreased over 20 years, and protection and immune memory persist in these children and young adults [83, 84].

There are few data on immunogenicity in children vaccinated after infancy. Eighty seven percent of Alaskan children vaccinated after 6 months of age were protected against infection for up to 22 years [85].

At this time, there is no specific recommendation from the CDC regarding booster vaccination, unless the anti-HBs titer, checked for the above indications or any other indication, is above 0 but less than 10 mIU/mL. In this situation, a single booster vaccination should be administered. If the anti-HBs titer is 0, the entire three-dose series should be repeated.

Adverse Reactions

Hepatitis B vaccines are extremely safe and well tolerated [86, 87]. The most common reactions are local, such as pain at the site of injection in 20%. Low-grade fever occurs in less than 5% of recipients. Anaphylaxis is extremely rare, but has been reported [88].

In the first few years following the development of the vaccine, there were reports of a possible association with Guillain–Barré syndrome (GBS) in adults who had received plasma-derived vaccine [89]. However, after thorough investigation from 1986 to 1990 by the CDC, FDA, and vaccine manufacturers, it was ascertained that the rate of GBS did not exceed that in unvaccinated adults. Therefore, clinical position papers concluded that a direct cause–effect relationship could not be refuted or accepted [90, 91].

In the late 1990s, there was debate regarding a causal relationship between HBV vaccines and multiple sclerosis [92]. This association was clearly and conclusively disproven by several studies [93, 94].

In 1999, concern was raised that thimerosal, a vaccine preservative, might cause mercury poisoning in young infants, although no cases were detected. However, given this apprehension, thimerosal-free vaccines were produced. While the new preparations were awaited, vaccines were withheld from infants unless they were born to HBV-infected mothers. By 2000, thimerosal-free preparations were available, but it took years to return to the immunization rates that had been achieved prior to 1999 [95]. One study demonstrated a sixfold increase in the number of hospitals not vaccinating all high-risk infants [96], although no cases of injury from thimerosal had been documented.

Preexposure Prophylaxis (Table 4)

Immunization policies regarding infants, children, and adolescents have evolved since the 1991 ACIP of the CDC made five major recommendations, but these are still the mainstays of the strategy developed to decrease the childhood burden of HBV [97]:

1. Screening all pregnant women for HBsAg;
2. Administration of HBIG and HBV vaccine within 12 h to babies born to HBsAg-seropositive mothers;

Table 4 Immunoprophylaxis summary for hepatitis B [51, 115]

Preexposure prophylaxis	
0–19 years	Hepatitis B vaccine series
Postexposure prophylaxis	
Perinatal exposure	HBIG and vaccine series
Mucosal/percutaneous	
Known titer ≥ 10 mIU/mL	No intervention
Immunized, low/no titer	Hepatitis B vaccine single dose
Unvaccinated	HBIG and vaccine series

HBIG hepatitis B immune globulin

3. Administration of vaccine within 12 h of birth to infants of untested mothers;
4. Universal immunization of babies born to HBsAg-negative mothers;
5. Vaccination of high-risk adolescents and adults.

Since that time, the final recommendation has been broadened to include vaccination of all children aged 0–18 years.

Studies in the USA have shown improved rates of universal vaccination for children during the first years, with an estimated 94% of children aged 19–35 months receiving the three-part series [98]. However, administration of the first dose of HBV vaccine at birth is still somewhat problematic, with only 55% of infants receiving vaccine in the first 3 days of life [98]. Vaccination of adolescents has still been an issue, with a lower immunization rate in older adolescents [99, 100].

Nonetheless, hepatitis B vaccination programs have been extremely successful in decreasing both acute and chronic hepatitis B in the USA and other parts of the world. In the USA, the incidence of acute hepatitis B among children aged <15 years has declined 98%, from 1.2 cases per 100,000 population in 1990 to 0.02 cases per 100,000 population in 2007 [1]. China has documented a 90% reduction in the prevalence of chronic hepatitis B in childhood, down to 1% of children less than 5 years of age [101].

As a result of decreasing the prevalence of chronic infection, HBV vaccination has also been shown to decrease the incidence of hepatocellular carcinoma (HCC). Studies from Taiwan have demonstrated a significant decrease in HCC incidence: from 0.70 per 100,000 children prevaccine (1981–1986), to 0.57 from 1986 to 1990, and 0.36 from 1990 to 1994 [102]. A recent 20-year follow-up of vaccinated children has confirmed these data, demonstrating the efficacy of HCC prevention into early adulthood [103].

Postexposure Prophylaxis (Table 4)

Perinatal Exposure

Both the HBV vaccine and HBIG must be administered within 12 h of birth to infants born to HBsAg-positive mothers, and the three-dose vaccine series needs to be completed. If the infant is premature and <2,000 g, vaccine should still be given, although it should not count toward the three-dose series. In most series, the combination of HBV vaccine and HBIG is 85–95% effective in preventing acute or chronic hepatitis B in infants at risk [104–106]. One recent study has documented the efficacy of this strategy as greater than 99% [107]. However, some reports from Asian populations have documented much higher HBV transmission rates (25–30%), even with the use of active and passive immunoprophylaxis, with greater risk attributed to high maternal viral load [108]. Because of this, alternative strategies using antiviral agents and administration of HBIG to affected mothers during the third trimester have been tested [108–110]. For example, lamivudine supplied to mothers in late pregnancy, in addition to HBV vaccine/HBIG at birth, has been shown to decrease transmission [108, 109]. At the present time, established guidelines recommend consideration of antiviral agents in the third trimester for highly viremic women who have previously transmitted hepatitis B to their newborns.

If maternal HBsAg status in unknown, vaccine should be given, and maternal HBsAg status should be tested within 7 days, as HBIG must be given within that time period [51].

In areas of the world where HBIG is either not available or too expensive, HBV vaccine is the only perinatal prophylaxis provided, with prevention rates of 70–95% [111–113].

The CDC recommends that infants born to HBsAg-positive mothers be tested for anti-HBs and HBsAg at 6–12 months after vaccination is completed. If the child is HBsAg negative, but the anti-HBs titer not ≥10 mIU/mL, the vaccination series should be repeated [51]. Even with proper implementation of this strategy, there is at least a 5% of perinatal HBV transmission. This rate may be higher if maternal viremia levels are very high. Some investigators advocate the use of antiviral medications in this setting, in addition to the immunoprophylaxis, but this is not yet part of standard obstetrical management. Infants identified as infected by this testing at 9–18 months of age should be referred for appropriate monitoring and management.

Mucosal or Percutaneous Exposure

Persons who have completed the three-dose vaccine series and have documented anti-HBs titer of ≥10 mIU/mL do not require prophylaxis if they are subsequently exposed to HBV through mucosal or percutaneous exposure. If a person completed the vaccination series, but never had a titer tested, an additional HBV vaccine dose should be administered, preferably within 24 h of exposure. Those persons who are unvaccinated and have sexual, mucosal, or percutaneous exposure should receive the combination of HBV vaccine and HBIG (0.06 mL/kg) intramuscularly within 24 h [114, 115].

Special Circumstances

Chemoprophylaxis with Transplantation or Immunosuppression

Although it is rare for children with chronic HBV to require liver transplantation, the recurrence rate would be expected to be high, and universal without intervention.

The use of HBIG in combination with lamivudine or adefovir dipivoxil has been well described in adults in this setting [116]. HBsAg-positive patients, with or without liver disease or active viral replication, are at risk of hepatic flares during immunosuppressive regimens for other solid organ or stem cell transplants [117–120]. In addition, major hepatic flares have occurred in HBV-infected individuals who require other immunosuppression, such as tumor necrosis factor-alpha antagonists or cancer chemotherapy [121, 122].

Even children with previous HBV infection (HBsAg negative, hepatitis B core antibody positive) are at risk of reactivation during hematopoietic stem cell or solid organ transplantation [123, 124]. Evaluation prior to transplant for evidence of previous or chronic HBV infection is indicated. Lamivudine or other nucleoside/nucleotide analog prophylaxis prior to and after transplant should be considered in this patient population [123].

Other children who may require lamivudine or other antiviral agents include HBsAg-negative patients who receive liver transplants from hepatitis B core antibody-positive donors [125] or stem cell transplant recipients who are HBV negative, but have HBV-positive donors [126]. In the latter situation, both donors and recipients have been treated with antivirals before and after transplantation [126].

Adoptive transfer of HBV immunity (anti-HBs) from donor to recipient has been documented through hematopoietic stem cell transplants [127]. In addition, there are case reports of antiviral therapy followed by successful adoptive transfer of anti-HBs through transplant, and subsequent HBsAg seroconversion and viral clearance from the HBV-infected recipient [128, 129].

Conclusions

Since the production of the HBV vaccine, the incidence of acute and chronic hepatitis B infections has been dramatically reduced in the USA and other parts of the world. Expanded immunization recommendations have stimulated even more progress in prevention of HBV infection. The vaccines are safe and extremely immunogenic. Vaccine should still be used in combination with HBIG for perinatally exposed infants, unvaccinated older children and adolescents with known recent exposure to hepatitis B, and cirrhotic patients undergoing transplantation. Further goals should be wider immunization of adolescents and adults, as well as improved vaccination rates in the first few days of life, especially in infants born to an HBsAg-positive or status unknown mothers.

References

1. Centers for Disease and Control and Prevention. Surveillance for acute viral hepatitis – United States, 2007. *MMWR Morb Mortal Wkly Rep.* 2009;58(SS-3).
2. American Academy of Pediatrics. Hepatitis A. In: Pickering LK, Baker CJ, Kimberlin DW, Long SS, eds. *2009 Red Book: Report of the Committee on Infectious Diseases.* Elk Grove Village, IL: American Academy of Pediatrics; 2009:329–337.

3. Hutin YJ, Sabin KM, Hutwagner LC, et al. Multiple modes of hepatitis A virus transmission among methamphetamine users. *Am J Epidemiol.* 2000;152(2):186–192.
4. Vong S, Fiore AE, Haight DO, et al. Vaccination in the county jail as a strategy to reach high risk adults during a community-based hepatitis A outbreak among methamphetamine drug users. *Vaccine.* 2005;23(8):1021–1028.
5. Cohn EJ, Oncley JL, Strong LE, Hughes WL, Armstrong SH. Chemical, clinical, and immunological studies on the products of human plasma fractionation. I. The characterization of the protein fractions of human plasma. *J Clin Invest.* 1944;23(4):417–432.
6. Centers for Disease and Control and Prevention. Prevention of hepatitis A through active or passive immunization: recommendations of the Advisory Committee on Immunization Practices (ACIP). *MMWR Morb Mortal Wkly Rep.* 2006;55(RR-7):1–23.
7. Stokes J Jr, Neefe JR. The prevention and attenuation of infectious hepatitis by gamma globulin: preliminary note. *JAMA.* 1945;127:144–145.
8. Ellis EF, Henney CS. Adverse reactions following administration of human gamma globulin. *J Allergy.* 1969;43(1):45–54.
9. Centers for Disease and Control and Prevention. General recommendations on immunization; recommendations of the Advisory Committee on Immunization Practices (ACIP) and the American Academy of Family Physicians (AAFP). *MMWR Morb Mortal Wkly Rep.* 2002;51(RR-2):1–36.
10. Centers for Disease and Control and Prevention. Prevention of varicella: recommendations of the Advisory Committee on Immunization Practices (ACIP). *MMWR Morb Mortal Wkly Rep.* 1996;45(RR-11):1–25.
11. Innis BL, Snitbhan R, Kunasol P, et al. Protection against hepatitis A by an inactivated vaccine. *JAMA.* 1994;271(17):1328–1334.
12. Werzberger A, Mensch B, Kuter B, et al. A controlled trial of a formalin-inactivated hepatitis A vaccine in healthy children. *N Engl J Med.* 1992;327(7):453–457.
13. Peetermans J. Production, quality control and characterization of an inactivated hepatitis A vaccine. *Vaccine.* 1992;10 Suppl 1:S99–S101.
14. Armstrong ME, Giesa PA, Davide JP, et al. Development of the formalin-inactivated hepatitis A vaccine, VAQTA from the live attenuated virus strain CR326F. *J Hepatol.* 1993;18 Suppl 2:S20–S26.
15. VAQTA Prescribing Information. 2007; Merck & Co., Inc. Website. Available at: http://www.merck.com.
16. McMahon BJ, Williams J, Bulkow L, et al. Immunogenicity of an inactivated hepatitis A vaccine in Alaska native children and native and non-native adults. *J Infect Dis.* 1995;171(3): 676–679.
17. Horng YC, Chang MH, Lee CY, et al. Safety and immunogenicity of hepatitis A vaccine in healthy children. *Pediatr Infect Dis J.* 1993;12(5):359–362.
18. Balcarek KB, Bagley MR, Pass RF, Schiff ER, Krause DS. Safety and immunogenicity of an inactivated hepatitis A vaccine in preschool children. *J Infect Dis.*1995;171 Suppl 1:S70–S72.
19. Ashur Y, Adler R, Rowe M, Shouval D. Comparison of immunogenicity of two hepatitis A vaccines – VAQTA and HAVRIX – in young adults. *Vaccine.* 1999;17(18):2290–2296.
20. Letson GW, Shapiro CN, Kuehn D, et al. Effect of maternal antibody on immunogenicity of hepatitis A vaccine in infants. *J Pediatr.* 2004;144(3):327–332.
21. Dagan R, Amir J, Mijalovsky A, et al. Immunization against hepatitis A in the first year of life: priming despite the presence of maternal antibody. *Pediatr Infect Dis J.* 2000;19(11): 1045–1052.
22. Lieberman JM, Chang SJ, Partridge S, et al. Kinetics of maternal hepatitis a antibody decay in infants: implications for vaccine use. *Pediatr Infect Dis J.* 2002;21(4):347–348.
23. Bell BP, Negus S, Fiore AE, et al. Immunogenicity of an inactivated hepatitis A vaccine in infants and young children. *Pediatr Infect Dis J.* 2007;26(2):116–122.
24. Gouvea AF, De Moraes-Pinto MI, Ono E, et al. Immunogenicity and tolerability of hepatitis A vaccine in HIV-infected children. *Clin Infect Dis.* 2005;41(4):544–548.
25. Siberry GK, Coller RJ, Henkle E, et al. Antibody response to hepatitis A immunization among human immunodeficiency virus-infected children and adolescents. *Pediatr Infect Dis J.* 2008;27(5):465–468.

26. Weinberg A, Gona P, Nachman SA, et al. Antibody responses to hepatitis A virus vaccine in HIV-infected children with evidence of immunologic reconstitution while receiving highly active antiretroviral therapy. *J Infect Dis*. 2006;193(2):302–311.
27. Arslan M, Wiesner RH, Poterucha JJ, Zein NN. Safety and efficacy of hepatitis A vaccination in liver transplantation recipients. *Transplantation*. 2001;72(2):272–276.
28. Diana A, Posfay-Barbe KM, Belli DC, Siegrist CA. Vaccine-induced immunity in children after orthotopic liver transplantation: a 12-yr review of the Swiss national reference center. *Pediatr Transplant*. 2007;11(1):31–37.
29. Gunther M, Stark K, Neuhaus R, et al. Rapid decline of antibodies after hepatitis A immunization in liver and renal transplant recipients. *Transplantation*. 2001;71(3):477–479.
30. Centers for Disease and Control and Prevention. Guidelines for preventing opportunistic infections among hematopoietic stem cell transplant recipients. *MMWR Recomm Rep*. 2000;49(RR-10):1–125, CE121-127.
31. Molrine DC. Recommendations for immunizations in stem cell transplantation. *Pediatr Transplant*. 2003;7 Suppl 3:76–85.
32. Keeffe EB, Iwarson S, McMahon BJ, et al. Safety and immunogenicity of hepatitis A vaccine in patients with chronic liver disease. *Hepatology*. 1998;27(3):881–886.
33. Ferreira CT, da Silveira TR, Vieira SM, et al. Immunogenicity and safety of hepatitis A vaccine in children with chronic liver disease. *J Pediatr Gastroenterol Nutr*. 2003;37(3):258–261.
34. El-Karaksy HM, El-Hawary MI, El-Koofy NM, et al. Safety and efficacy of hepatitis A vaccine in children with chronic liver disease. *World J Gastroenterol*. 2006;12(45):7337–7340.
35. Majda-Stanislawska E, Bednarek M, Kuydowicz J. Immunogenicity of inactivated hepatitis A vaccine in children with chronic liver disease. *Pediatr Infect Dis J*. 2004;23(6):571–574.
36. Hammitt LL, Bulkow L, Hennessy TW, et al. Persistence of antibody to hepatitis A virus 10 years after vaccination among children and adults. *J Infect Dis*. 2008;198(12): 1776–1782.
37. Werzberger A, Mensch B, Nalin DR, Kuter BJ. Effectiveness of hepatitis A vaccine in a former frequently affected community: 9 years' followup after the Monroe field trial of VAQTA. *Vaccine*. 2002;20(13–14):1699–1701.
38. Werzberger A, Mensch B, Taddeo C, et al. 6-year follow up of children and adolescents who participated in an efficacy trial of VAQTA (hepatitis A vaccine, inactivated, Merck). *Conference abstracts of the 32nd National Immunization Conference*. Atlanta, GA: US Department of Health and Human Services, CDC; 1998.
39. Centers for Disease and Control and Prevention. Prevention of hepatitis A through active or passive immunization: recommendations of the Advisory Committee on Immunization Practices (ACIP). *MMWR Recomm Rep*. 1999;48(RR-12):1–37.
40. Wasley A, Samandari T, Bell BP. Incidence of hepatitis A in the United States in the era of vaccination. *JAMA*. 2005;294(2):194–201.
41. Centers for Disease and Control and Prevention. Update: Prevention of hepatitis A after exposure to hepatitis A virus and in international travelers. Updated recommendations of the Advisory Committee on Immunization Practices (ACIP). *MMWR Morb Mortal Wkly Rep*. 2007;56(41):1080–1084.
42. Centers for Disease and Control and Prevention. Updated recommendations from the Advisory Committee on Immunization Practices (ACIP) for use of hepatitis A vaccine in close contacts of newly arriving international adoptees. *MMWR Morb Mortal Wkly Rep*. 2009;58(36):1006–1007.
43. Cotter SM, Sansom S, Long T, et al. Outbreak of hepatitis A among men who have sex with men: implications for hepatitis A vaccination strategies. *J Infect Dis*. 2003;187(8):1235–1240.
44. Dienstag JL, Davenport FM, McCollum RW, et al. Nonhuman primate-associated viral hepatitis type A. Serologic evidence of hepatitis A virus infection. *JAMA*. 1976;236(5): 462–464.
45. Centers for Disease and Control and Prevention. Blood safety monitoring among persons with bleeding disorders – United States, May 1998-June 2002. *MMWR Morb Mortal Wkly Rep*. 2003;51(51–52):1152–1154.
46. Mosley JW, Reisler DM, Brachott D, et al. Comparison of two lots of immune serum globulin for prophylaxis of infectious hepatitis. *Am J Epidemiol*. 1968;87(3):539–550.

47. Sagliocca L, Amoroso P, Stroffolini T, et al. Efficacy of hepatitis A vaccine in prevention of secondary hepatitis A infection: a randomised trial. *Lancet.* 1999;353(9159):1136–1139.
48. Sagliocca L, Bianco E, Amoroso P, et al. Feasibility of vaccination in preventing secondary cases of hepatitis A virus infection. *Vaccine.* 2005;23(7):910–914.
49. Victor JC, Monto AS, Surdina TY, et al. Hepatitis A vaccine versus immune globulin for postexposure prophylaxis. *N Engl J Med.* 2007;357(17):1685–1694.
50. McMahon BJ, Alward WLM, Hall DB, et al. Acute hepatitis B virus infection: relation of age to the clinical expression of disease and subsequent development of the carrier state. *J Infect Dis.* 1985;151:599–603.
51. Mast EE, Margolis HS, Fiore AE, et al. A comprehensive immunization strategy to eliminate transmission of hepatitis B virus infection in the United States: recommendations of the Advisory Committee on Immunization Practices (ACIP) part 1: immunization of infants, children, and adolescents. *Recomm Rep.* 2005;54(RR-16):1–31.
52. Emini EA, Ellis RW, Miller WJ, et al. Production and immunological analysis of recombinant hepatitis B vaccine. *J Infect.* 1986;13 Suppl A:3–9.
53. Bush LM, Moonsammy GI, Boscia JA. Evaluation of initiating a hepatitis B vaccination schedule with one vaccine and completing it with another. *Vaccine.* 1991;9(11):807–809.
54. Goldfarb J, Baley J, Medendorp SV, et al. Comparative study of the immunogenicity and safety of two dosing schedules of Engerix-B hepatitis B vaccine in neonates. *Pediatr Infect Dis J.* 1994;13(1):18–22.
55. Greenberg DP. Pediatric experience with recombinant hepatitis B vaccines and relevant safety and immunogenicity studies. *Pediatr Infect Dis J.* 1993;12(5):438–445.
56. Greenberg DP, Vadheim CM, Marcy SM, et al. Safety and immunogenicity of a recombinant hepatitis B vaccine administered to infants at 2, 4 and 6 months of age. The Kaiser-UCLA Vaccine Study Group. *Vaccine.* 1996;14(8):811–816.
57. Greenberg DP, Vadheim CM, Wong VK, et al. Comparative safety and immunogenicity of two recombinant hepatitis B vaccines given to infants at two, four and six months of age. *Pediatr Infect Dis J.* 1996;15(7):590–596.
58. Nemes E, Lefler E, Szegedi L, et al. Gluten intake interferes with the humoral immune response to recombinant hepatitis B vaccine in patients with celiac disease. *Pediatrics.* 2008; 121(6):e1570–e1576.
59. Leonardi S, Spina M, Spicuzza L, Rotolo N, La Rosa M. Hepatitis B vaccination failure in celiac disease: is there a need to reassess current immunization strategies? *Vaccine.* 2009;27(43):6030–6033.
60. Weber DJ, Rutala WA, Samsa GP, Santimaw JE, Lemon SM. Obesity as a predictor of poor antibody response to hepatitis B plasma vaccine. *JAMA.* 1985;254(22):3187–3189.
61. Middleman AB, Anding R, Tung C. Effect of needle length when immunizing obese adolescents with hepatitis B vaccine. *Pediatrics.* 2010;125:e508–e512.
62. Lau YL, Tam AY, Ng KW, et al. Response of preterm infants to hepatitis B vaccine. *J Pediatr.* 1992;121(6):962–965.
63. Linder N, Vishne TH, Levin E, et al. Hepatitis B vaccination: long-term follow-up of the immune response of preterm infants and comparison of two vaccination protocols. *Infection.* 2002;30(3):136–139.
64. Losonsky GA, Wasserman SS, Stephens I, et al. Hepatitis B vaccination of premature infants: a reassessment of current recommendations for delayed immunization. *Pediatrics.* 1999;103(2):E14.
65. Huang FY, Li PI, Lee CY, Huang LM, Chang LY, Liu SC. Hepatitis B vaccination in preterm infants. *Arch Dis Child.* 1997;99:534–536.
66. Kim SC, Chung EK, Hodinka RL, et al. Immunogenicity of hepatitis B vaccine in preterm infants. *Pediatrics.* 1997;99(4):534–536.
67. Drachman R, Isacsohn M, Rudensky B, Drukker A. Vaccination against hepatitis B in children and adolescent patients on dialysis. *Nephrol Dial Transplant.* 1989;4(5):372–374.
68. Watkins SL, Alexander SR, Brewer ED, et al. Response to recombinant hepatitis B vaccine in children and adolescents with chronic renal failure. *Am J Kidney Dis.* 2002;40(2):365–372.

69. Vazquez G, Mendoza-Guevara L, Alvarez T, et al. Comparison of the response to the recombinant vaccine against hepatitis B virus in dialyzed and nondialyzed children with CRF using different doses and routes of administration. *Adv Perit Dial.* 1997;13:291–296.
70. Wilson CM, Ellenberg JH, Sawyer MK, et al. Serologic response to hepatitis B vaccine in HIV infected and high-risk HIV uninfected adolescents in the REACH cohort. Reaching for Excellence in Adolescent Care and Health. *J Adolesc Health.* 2001;29(3 Suppl):123–129.
71. Zuin G, Principi N, Tornaghi R, et al. Impaired response to hepatitis B vaccine in HIV infected children. *Vaccine.* 1992;10(12):857–860.
72. Simani OE, Leroux-Roels G, Francois G, Burnett RJ, Meheus A, Mphahlele MJ. Reduced detection and levels of protective antibodies to hepatitis B vaccine in under 2-year-old HIV positive South African children at a paediatric outpatient clinic. *Vaccine.* 2009;27(1):146–151.
73. Abzug MJ, Warshaw M, Rosenblatt HM, et al. Immunogenicity and immunologic memory after hepatitis B virus booster vaccination in HIV-infected children receiving highly active antiretroviral therapy. *J Infect Dis.* 2009;200(6):935–946.
74. Meral A, Sevinir B, Gunay U. Efficacy of immunization against hepatitis B virus infection in children with cancer. *Med Pediatr Oncol.* 2000;35(1):47–51.
75. Polychronopoulou-Androulakaki S, Panagiotou JP, Kostaridou S, Kyratzopoulou A, Haidas S. Immune response of immunocompromised children with malignancies to a recombinant hepatitis B vaccine. *Pediatr Hematol Oncol.* 1996;13(5):425–431.
76. Jaffe D, Papadopoulos EB, Young JW, et al. Immunogenicity of recombinant hepatitis B vaccine (rHBV) in recipients of unrelated or related allogeneic hematopoietic cell (HC) transplants. *Blood.* 2006;108(7):2470–2475.
77. Loinaz C, de Juanes JR, Gonzalez EM, et al. Hepatitis B vaccination results in 140 liver transplant recipients. *Hepatogastroenterology.* 1997;44(13):235–238.
78. Petersen KM, Bulkow LR, McMahon BJ, et al. Duration of hepatitis B immunity in low risk children receiving hepatitis B vaccinations from birth. *Pediatr Infect Dis J.* 2004;23(7):650–655.
79. Lin YC, Chang MH, Ni YH, Hsu HY, Chen DS. Long-term immunogenicity and efficacy of universal hepatitis B virus vaccination in Taiwan. *J Infect Dis.* 2003;187(1):134–138.
80. Lu CY, Chiang BL, Chi WK, et al. Waning immunity to plasma-derived hepatitis B vaccine and the need for boosters 15 years after neonatal vaccination. *Hepatology.* 2004;40(6):1415–1420.
81. Yuen MF, Lim WL, Cheng CC, Lam SK, Lai CL. Twelve-year follow-up of a prospective randomized trial of hepatitis B recombinant DNA yeast vaccine versus plasma-derived vaccine without booster doses in children. *Hepatology.* 1999;29(3):924–927.
82. Yuen MF, Lim WL, Chan AO, Wong DK, Sum SS, Lai CL. 18-year follow-up study of a prospective randomized trial of hepatitis B vaccinations without booster doses in children. *Clin Gastroenterol Hepatol.* 2004;2(10):941–945.
83. van der Sande MA, Waight P, Mendy M, et al. Long-term protection against carriage of hepatitis B virus after infant vaccination. *J Infect Dis.* 2006;193(11):1528–1535.
84. But DY, Lai CL, Lim WL, Fung J, Wong DK, Yuen MF. Twenty-two years follow-up of a prospective randomized trial of hepatitis B vaccines without booster dose in children: final report. *Vaccine.* 2008;26(51):6587–6591.
85. McMahon BJ, Dentinger CM, Bruden D, et al. Antibody levels and protection after hepatitis B vaccine: results of a 22-year follow-up study and response to a booster dose. *J Infect Dis.* 2009;200(9):1390–1396.
86. Andre FE. Summary of safety and efficacy data on a yeast-derived hepatitis B vaccine. *Am J Med.* 1989;87(3):14S–20S.
87. Zajac BA, West DJ, McAleer WJ, Scolnick EM. Overview of clinical studies with hepatitis B vaccine made by recombinant DNA. *J Infect.* 1986;13 Suppl A:39–45.
88. Bohlke K, Davis RL, Marcy SM, et al. Risk of anaphylaxis after vaccination of children and adolescents. *Pediatrics.* 2003;112(4):815–820.
89. Shaw FE, Jr., Graham DJ, Guess HA, et al. Postmarketing surveillance for neurologic adverse events reported after hepatitis B vaccination. Experience of the first three years. *Am J Epidemiol.* 1988;127(2):337–352.

90. Stratton KR, Howe CJ, Johnston RB, Jr. Adverse events associated with childhood vaccines other than pertussis and rubella. Summary of a report from the Institute of Medicine. *JAMA.* 1994;271(20):1602–1605.
91. Centers for Disease and Control and Prevention. Update: vaccine side effects, adverse reactions, contraindications, and precautions. Recommendations of the Advisory Committee on Immunization Practices (ACIP). *MMWR Recomm Rep.*1996;45(RR-12):1–35.
92. Hernan MA, Jick SS, Olek MJ, Jick H. Recombinant hepatitis B vaccine and the risk of multiple sclerosis: a prospective study. *Neurology.*2004;63(5):838–842.
93. Ascherio A, Zhang SM, Hernan MA, et al. Hepatitis B vaccination and the risk of multiple sclerosis. *N Engl J Med.* 2001;344(5):327–332.
94. Halsey NA, Van Duclos P, Damme P, Margolis H. Hepatitis vaccine and central nervous system demyelinating diseases. Viral Hepatitis Prevention Board. *Pediatr Infect Dis J.* 1999;18(1):23–24.
95. Luman ET, Fiore AE, Strine TW, Barker LE. Impact of thimerosal-related changes in hepatitis B vaccine birth-dose recommendations on childhood vaccination coverage. *JAMA.* 2004;291(19):2351–2358.
96. Clark S, Cabana M, Malik T, Yusuf H, Freed G. Hepatitis B vaccination practices in hospital newborn nurseries before and after changes in vaccination recommendations. *Arch Pediatr Adolesc Med.* 2001;155:915–920.
97. Centers for Disease and Control and Prevention. Update: recommendations to prevent hepatitis B virus transmission – United States. *MMWR Morb Mortal Wkly Rep.* 1999;48(2):33–34.
98. Centers for Disease and Control and Prevention. National, state, and local area vaccination coverage among children aged 19–35 months – United States, 2008. *MMWR Morb Mortal Wkly Rep.* 2009;58(33):921–926.
99. Gonzalez IM, Averhoff FM, Massoudi MS, et al. Hepatitis B vaccination among adolescents in 3 large health maintenance organizations. *Pediatrics.* 2002;110(5):929–934.
100. Jain N, Hennessey K. Hepatitis B vaccination coverage among U.S. adolescents, National Immunization Survey-Teen, 2006. *J Adolesc Health.* 2009;44(6):561–567.
101. Liang X, Bi S, Yang W, et al. Epidemiological serosurvey of hepatitis B in China – declining HBV prevalence due to hepatitis B vaccination. *Vaccine.* 2009;27(47):6550–6557.
102. Chang MH, Chen CJ, Lai MS, et al. Universal hepatitis B vaccination in Taiwan and the incidence of hepatocellular carcinoma in children. Taiwan Childhood Hepatoma Study Group. *N Engl J Med.* 1997;336:1906–1907.
103. Chang MH, You SL, Chen CJ, et al. Decreased incidence of hepatocellular carcinoma in hepatitis B vaccinees: a 20-year follow-up study. *J Natl Cancer Inst.* 2009;101(19):1348–1355.
104. Beasley RP, Hwang LY, Lee GC, et al. Prevention of perinatally transmitted hepatitis B virus infections with hepatitis B virus infections with hepatitis B immune globulin and hepatitis B vaccine. *Lancet.* 1983;2(8359):1099–1102.
105. Wong VC, Ip HM, Reesink HW, et al. Prevention of the HBsAg carrier state in newborn infants of mothers who are chronic carriers of HBsAg and HBeAg by administration of hepatitis-B vaccine and hepatitis-B immunoglobulin. Double-blind randomised placebo-controlled study. *Lancet.* 1984;1(8383):921–926.
106. Stevens CE, Taylor PE, Tong MJ, et al. Yeast-recombinant hepatitis B vaccine. Efficacy with hepatitis B immune globulin in prevention of perinatal hepatitis B virus transmission. *JAMA.* 1987;257(19):2612–2616.
107. Boot HJ, Hahne S, Cremer J, Wong A, Boland G, van Loon AM. Persistent and transient hepatitis B virus (HBV) infections in children born to HBV-infected mothers despite active and passive vaccination. *J Viral Hepat.* December 2009. doi. 10.1111/j.1365-2893.2009.01247.x.
108. Xu WM, Cui YT, Wang L, et al. Lamivudine in late pregnancy to prevent perinatal transmission of hepatitis B virus infection: a multicentre, randomized, double-blind, placebo-controlled study. *J Viral Hepat.* 2009;16(2):94–103.
109. van Zonneveld M, van Nunen AB, Niesters HG, de Man RA, Schalm SW, Janssen HL. Lamivudine treatment during pregnancy to prevent perinatal transmission of hepatitis B virus infection. *J Viral Hepat.* 2003;10(4):294–297.

110. Xiao XM, Li AZ, Chen X, Zhu YK, Miao J. Prevention of vertical hepatitis B transmission by hepatitis B immunoglobulin in the third trimester of pregnancy. *Int J Gynaecol Obstet.* 2007;96(3):167–170.
111. Hsu HM, Chen DS, Chuang CH, et al. Efficacy of a mass hepatitis B vaccination program in Taiwan. Studies on 3464 infants of hepatitis B surface antigen-carrier mothers. *JAMA.* 1988;260(15):2231–2235.
112. Milne A, West DJ, Chinh DV, Moyes CD, Poerschke G. Field evaluation of the efficacy and immunogenicity of recombinant hepatitis B vaccine without HBIG in newborn Vietnamese infants. *J Med Virol.* 2002;67(3):327–333.
113. Lolekha S, Warachit B, Hirunyachote A, Bowonkiratikachorn P, West DJ, Poerschke G. Protective efficacy of hepatitis B vaccine without HBIG in infants of HBeAg-positive carrier mothers in Thailand. *Vaccine.* 2002;20(31–32):3739–3743.
114. Centers for Disease and Control and Prevention. Updated U.S. Public Health Service guidelines for the management of occupational exposures to HBV, HCV, and HIV and recommendations for postexposure prophylaxis. *MMWR Recomm Rep.* 2001;50(RR-11):1–52.
115. Centers for Disease and Control and Prevention. Postexposure Prophylaxis to Prevent Hepatitis B Virus Infection. *MMWR Morb Mortal Wkly Rep.* 2006;55(RR 16 Appendix B):30–31.
116. Gish RG, McCashland T. Hepatitis B in liver transplant recipients. *Liver Transpl.* 2006;12(11 Suppl 2):S54–S64.
117. Hoofnagle JH. Reactivation of hepatitis B. *Hepatology.* 2009;49(5 Suppl):S156–S165.
118. Dusheiko G, Song E, Bowyer S, et al. Natural history of hepatitis B virus infection in renal transplant recipients – a fifteen-year follow-up. *Hepatology.*1983;3(3):330–336.
119. Degos F, Lugassy C, Degott C, et al. Hepatitis B virus and hepatitis B-related viral infection in renal transplant recipients. A prospective study of 90 patients. *Gastroenterology.* 1988;94(1):151–156.
120. Ko WJ, Chou NK, Hsu RB, et al. Hepatitis B virus infection in heart transplant recipients in a hepatitis B endemic area. *J Heart Lung Transplant.* 2001;20(8):865–875.
121. Papa A, Mocci G, Bonizzi M, et al. Use of infliximab in particular clinical settings: management based on current evidence. *Am J Gastroenterol.* 2009;104(6):1575–1586.
122. Mindikoglu AL, Regev A, Schiff ER. Hepatitis B virus reactivation after cytotoxic chemotherapy: the disease and its prevention. *Clin Gastroenterol Hepatol.* 2006;4(9):1076–1081.
123. Faraci M, Cappelli B, Lanino E, et al. Hepatitis B reactivation in allogeneic hemopoietic stem cell transplantation setting: a pediatric experience. *Pediatr Transplant.* 2009;13(7):923–926.
124. Knoll A, Pietrzyk M, Loss M, Goetz WA, Jilg W. Solid-organ transplantation in HBsAg-negative patients with antibodies to HBV core antigen: low risk of HBV reactivation. *Transplantation.* 2005;79(11):1631–1633.
125. Yu AS, Vierling JM, Colquhoun SD, et al. Transmission of hepatitis B infection from hepatitis B core antibody – positive liver allografts is prevented by lamivudine therapy. *Liver Transpl.* 2001;7(6):513–517.
126. Hui CK, Lie A, Au WY, et al. Effectiveness of prophylactic Anti-HBV therapy in allogeneic hematopoietic stem cell transplantation with HBsAg positive donors. *Am J Transplant.* 2005;5(6):1437–1445.
127. Lindemann M, Barsegian V, Runde V, et al. Transfer of humoral and cellular hepatitis B immunity by allogeneic hematopoietic cell transplantation. *Transplantation.* 2003;75(6):833–838.
128. Chiba T, Yokosuka O, Goto S, et al. Successful clearance of hepatitis B virus after allogeneic stem cell transplantation: beneficial combination of adoptive immunity transfer and lamivudine. *Eur J Haematol.* 2003;71(3):220–223.
129. Groll AH, Baumann-Kohler M, Storkebaum B, Kuhn J, Jurgens H, Vormoor J. Durable clearance of hepatitis B virus after allogeneic blood stem cell transplantation by adoptive immunity transfer and antiviral chemotherapy. *Pediatr Infect Dis J.* 2003;22(8):753–755.
130. Centers for Disease and Control and Prevention. Hepatitis A. *CDC Health Information for International Travel 2010.* Atlanta: U.S. Department of Health and Human Services, Public Health Service; 2009.

Primary Care of Children with Viral Hepatitis: Diagnosis, Monitoring, and General Management

Jessi Erlichman, Will Mellman, and Barbara A. Haber

Key Concepts

- Identification of children with hepatitis B or hepatitis C requires a heightened awareness of whom to screen, and which tests to obtain.
- Recent recommendations for hepatitis B case identification include screening of any person born in an area of the world where the prevalence exceeds 2%, or children born in the USA to parents who have emigrated from endemic regions.
- Chronic hepatitis B is a life-long disease that requires monitoring that is best managed as a partnership between the primary practitioner and the specialist.
- Vaccination is the best method of preventing hepatitis B transmission and titer measurement post-vaccination is recommended for close contacts.
- Like hepatitis B, hepatitis C in childhood frequently is undetected without knowing whom to screen.
- The best method of testing for hepatitis C is determination of antibody (anti-HCV).
- Children in whom HCV RNA is detected by PCR should be referred for consideration of treatment. Quantitative hepatitis C RNA and genotype testing are helpful in making treatment decisions and determining the likelihood of treatment response.
- Social aspects of both hepatitis B and C are essential areas of discussion for the practitioner, who should address alcohol use, illicit drugs, and sexual transmission.
- Family members of children with hepatitis B or hepatitis C should undergo appropriate testing and teaching about strategies to reduce transmission within the home.
- Children with hepatitis B or hepatitis C should not be excluded from school or extracurricular activities. Universal precautions that should already be in place in these settings are sufficient.

J. Erlichman (✉)
Division of GI and Nutrition, Children's Hospital of Philadelphia, 34th St & Civic Ctr Blvd, Philadelphia, PA 19104, USA
e-mail: haber@email.chop.edu

M.M. Jonas (ed.), *Viral Hepatitis in Children: Unique Features and Opportunities*, Clinical Gastroenterology, DOI 10.1007/978-1-60761-373-2_9,

Keywords Hepatitis B • Hepatitis C • Screening • Counseling • Vaccine • Immunization • Transmission • Treatment

Despite implementation of screening and vaccination programs, the global public health burden attributed to chronic hepatitis B virus (HBV) and hepatitis C virus (HCV) infections is staggering. In the USA, chronic viral hepatitis causes more deaths per year than human immunodeficiency (HIV) [1] and is a leading indication for liver transplantation in adults. The World Health Organization (WHO) estimates that 2 billion people have been infected with HBV and that 180 million people have been infected with HCV [2]. Although HBV is not endemic in the contiguous USA, rates of chronic infection have remained constant at 5% per 100,000 over the past 20 years, and in the USA, prevalence of chronic HCV infection is 1.8% and may, in fact, be significantly higher [3, 4]. It is incumbent upon the primary practitioner to understand that these diseases remain prevalent in the USA and that only with knowledge of whom to screen and how to screen will patients be identified and managed optimally. This chapter will focus on the screening and identification of chronic HBV and HCV infections in pediatrics and will provide clinical suggestions for monitoring and managing identified cases.

Hepatitis B

Natural History

Since 1981, the Centers for Disease Control and Prevention (CDC) has proposed a variety of recommendations to prevent the vertical and horizontal transmission of HBV. The current United States strategy for the prevention of HBV infection involves a complementary approach, incorporating universal immunization strategies combined with screening and identification of HBV-infected individuals or individuals at risk of infection. These strategies, however, are inconsistently implemented, and thus, chronic HBV infections persist among pediatric populations.

Worldwide, most cases of chronic hepatitis B are due to acquisition of the infection in childhood. Risk of developing chronic HBV infection is inversely related to age at the time of virus acquisition; of individuals who contract HBV infection as an infant, as a child <5 years, or as a child ≥5 years of age, 90, 30, and <5%, respectively, will develop chronic infection [5, 6]. Prior to the availability of the hepatitis B vaccine, an estimated 24,000 children contracted HBV infection each year in the USA [7] and adolescents were among the highest risk group. Now, however, universal childhood vaccination programs in the USA, combined with comprehensive perinatal screening programs, have significantly reduced the rate of newly acquired HBV infections, with the greatest decline among infants and children. Even with these measures, chronic HBV infection in the pediatric population remains prevalent.

Table 1 Geographic prevalence of chronic HBV infection

Geographic prevalence of chronic HBV infection (HbsAg)		
Low (<2%)	Intermediate (2–7%)	High (≤8%)
Australia	Areas surrounding Amazon River Basin	Caribbean (Haiti and Dominican Republic)
Canada (except Northern Territories)	Central America (Honduras and Guatemala)	Greenland
Mexico	Eastern and Southern Europe	Interior Amazon Basin
New Zealand	Israel	Middle East (except Israel)
Northern and Western Europe	Japan	Southeast Asia (China, Korea, Indonesia, and the Philippines)
Southern South American (Argentina and Chile)	Russia	South and Western Pacific Islands
United States (excluding Alaska and Hawaii)	Central, South, and Southwest Asia	Sub-Saharan Africa

The largest group of patients contributing to the continued presence of chronic HBV in the USA is persons born outside of the contiguous USA. Much of the world is still not vaccinated, and mandatory perinatal screening programs are unique to a select number of countries. Worldwide, the prevalence of chronic HBV infection ranges from high endemicity (>8%), to intermediate (2–8%) and low (<2%) [3] (Table 1); 75% of the world's population lives in areas characterized by a high rate of chronic infection. Although chronic HBV is not endemic in the contiguous USA, Alaska and Hawaii are characterized by high endemicity rates. The newest screening recommendations from the CDC include screening all international adoptees and any person born in geographic regions where hepatitis B surface antigen (HBsAg) prevalence is ≥2% [4]. Thus, screening of refugee, immigrant, or adopted children from high and intermediate HBV-endemic regions, despite asymptomatic appearance, is imperative.

While the CDC has implemented a comprehensive perinatal HBV screening program, vertically acquired HBV infections persist in the USA. Despite widely adopted prenatal screening in the USA, 61% of the estimated 23,000 women with infectious HBV who give birth each year are not identified through prenatal screening [8]. This gap in healthcare delivery is critical because in order to prevent vertical transmission, immunoprophylaxis with HBIG in conjunction with the first dose of the HBV vaccine must be administered to the neonate within 12–24 h of birth. When administered within this time frame, the protective efficacy is between 90 and 95%. A small percentage of infants are infected vertically even when all proper precautions are undertaken, including prenatal screening of the mother and institution of HBIG and vaccine in a timely manner. Up to 5% will acquire the infection either due to in utero acquisition or due to a high maternal viremia at the time of delivery. It is for that reason that it is recommended to test all children born to HBsAg-positive mothers around 12 months of age [4, 9].

Horizontal transmission, although less common than in previous decades, remains problematic. Infants who do not contract the virus from their carrier mothers during the perinatal period remain at risk for subsequent transmission during childhood. The household setting is a risk for horizontal transmission when HBV-infected persons do not take appropriate precautions. Individuals who are chronic HBV carriers pose the greatest risk for transmitting the virus to healthy contacts. Modes of transmission range from benign activities, such as sharing a toothbrush or razor, to percutaneous and permucosal exposure to infected body fluids. Studies suggest that the serologic prevalence of resolved HBV infection in households with persons with chronic HBV infection is 14–60%, and the prevalence of chronic infection amongst these unvaccinated household members is between 3 and 20% [10–13]. Therefore, children who cohabitate with known HBsAg-positive household members should be screened, as chronically infected individuals are the major reservoir for horizontal transmission. Despite vaccination, horizontal transmission can occur because not everyone develops protective titers. Universal recommendations for checking titers following vaccination do not exist; however, certain groups may need to demonstrate HBV immunity as a condition of employment or to attend school. Household contacts of HBsAg-positive people should also have titers checked to ensure HBV immunity.

In summary, the CDC updated screening recommendations suggest routine serologic testing with HBsAg for persons born in countries where prevalence of HBsAg exceeds 2%, regardless of the patient's vaccination status in their country of origin; infants born to mothers with unknown HBsAg or positive-HBsAg status; those with unexplained liver disease characterized by persistently elevated alanine aminotransferase (ALT) or asparate aminotransferase (AST) levels of unknown etiology; children born in the USA to parents who immigrated from endemic areas; persons receiving cytotoxic or immunosuppressive therapy; and persons with behavioral exposures to HBV, which may include people who reside in correctional facilities or who frequently travel to HBV-endemic regions of the world [4].

Screening and Diagnosis

Serologic testing with hepatitis B surface antigen (HBsAg) is the primary screening laboratory test to identify persons with hepatitis B infection, either acute or chronic. The only exception is in acute HBV, where there is effective resolution of HBsAg. In that situation, anti-HBs core IgM may be the only marker present during the so-called "window period." Identification of HBsAg in serum is indicative of HBV infection and, by law, must be reported to state and local health authorities in accordance with state reporting statutes. All patients with risk factors for HBV should be tested despite negative physical examination findings or normal or nonspecific laboratory test results. Most individuals with chronic HBV are asymptomatic; therefore, knowing whom to screen is key to identifying infected individuals. The interpretation of laboratory tests used for identifying a person's HBV status is provided in Fig. 1.

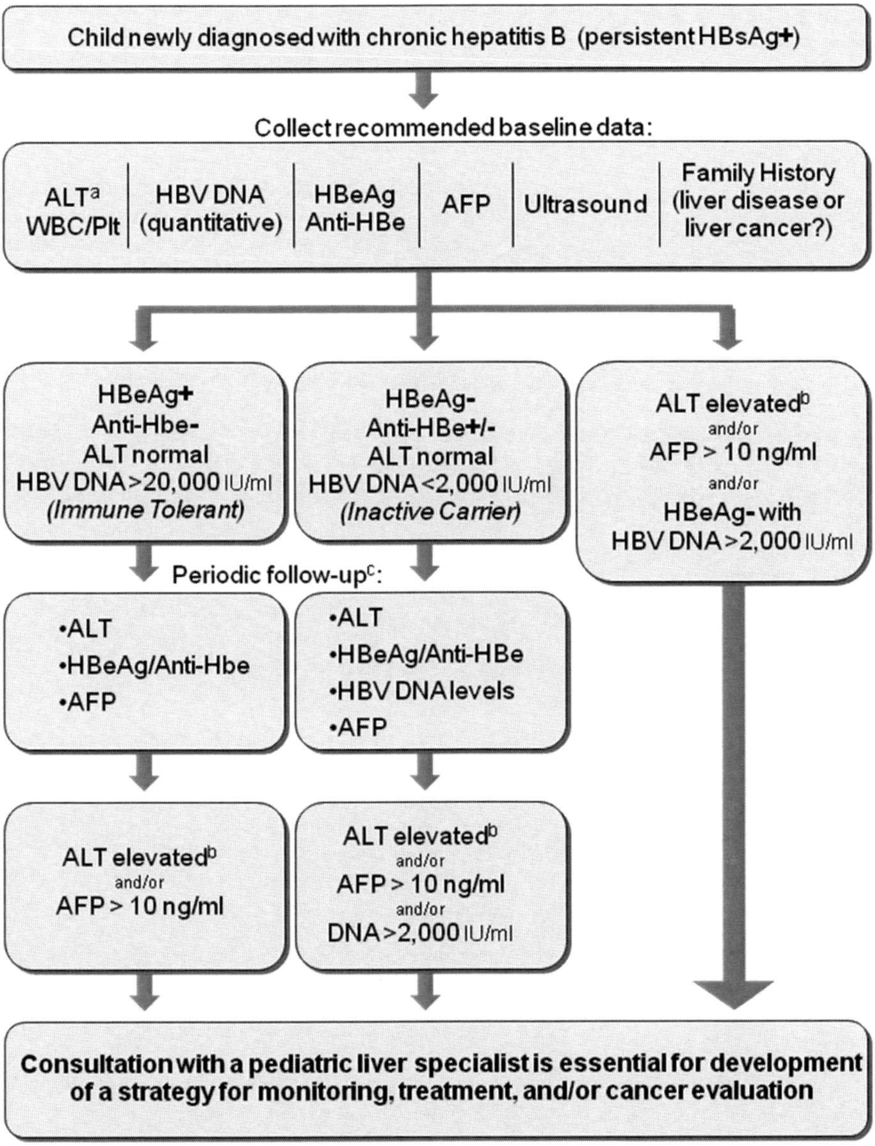

Fig. 1 Recommended approach to monitoring children with chronic hepatitis B infection. Reproduced with permission from *Pediatrics*, vol. 124, pages e1007–13, copyright ©2009 by the AAP

When a patient is identified as having chronic HBV infection, the initial evaluation should involve a physical examination with a thorough medical history. A comprehensive medical history must be obtained to identify risk factors for coinfections and disease progression, and to detail family history of HBV infection and/or liver cancer. Comprehensive laboratory testing should be undertaken to assess

Table 2 Hepatitis B and Hepatitis C viral tests

Viral hepatitis markers	
Hepatitis B	
Hepatitis B surface antigen (HBsAg)	Presence of this protein antigen in the blood indicates a person is infected with HBV
Hepatitis B surface antibody (anti-HBs)	Presence demonstrates immunity as a result of either vaccination or natural infection
Hepatitis B e antigen (HBeAg)	Presence of this viral protein reflects active viral replication and degree of infectivity, and can be used as a measure of treatment effectiveness
Hepatitis B e antibody (anti-HBe)	Indicates previous exposure to HBV, such as via vaccination, but the virus is no longer present and the person cannot pass the virus to others. Antibody presence protects the body from future HBV infection
Hepatitis B e antibody (anti-HBe) in the presence of HBsAg	Indicates reduced viral replication and possible inactive liver disease
Hepatitis B virus deoxyribonucleic acid (HBV DNA)	Presence reflects ongoing liver disease; patient is highly infectious
Hepatitis B core antibody (anti-HBc)	Indicates a person has recently been exposed to HBV and may or may not still be infected. Isolated results can lead to a false positive; therefore, this test is usually ordered in conjunction with other serologic markers
Immunoglobin M fraction of the hepatitis B core antibody (IgM anti-HBc)	Presence suggests recent infection with HBV
Hepatitis C	
Hepatitis C virus antibody (Anti-HCV)	Indicates past or present infection. Does not differentiate among acute, chronic, or past infections
Hepatitis C virus ribonucleic acid (HCV RNA) (qualitative)	Detects presence or absence of virus. More sensitive than quantitative PCR assays
Hepatitis C virus ribonucleic acid (HCV RNA) (quantitative)	Determines and quantifies viral load

liver disease status as measured by ALT level and white blood cell and platelet counts (measured as part of a complete blood count (CBC)); serologic markers of HBV replication (HBeAg, anti-HBe, HBV DNA); and testing to identify possible coinfection with HCV, HDV, or HIV. A summary of the significance of hepatitis B viral markers is provided in Table 2. All patients whose hepatitis A (HAV) immune status is unknown should receive two doses of the hepatitis A vaccine in the recommended schedule. Other clinical testing that may be warranted during an initial evaluation or over the course of follow-up includes baseline and periodic alfa-fetoprotein (AFP) assay to stratify risk of hepatocellular carcinoma (HCC), and ultrasound imaging to assess liver echotexture, nodules, and masses as well as spleen size.

Medical Management of Chronic Infection

In pediatric chronic HBV infection, the phase of infection is an important determinant for the risk of disease progression and likelihood of treatment response. There are four phases of chronic HBV infection and infected persons can evolve or revert from phase to phase. The four recognized phases are (1) the immune-tolerant phase, which is characterized by positive serum HBsAg and HBeAg, with high levels of HBV DNA (>20,000 IU/mL or 100,000 copies/mL) but absence of liver inflammation, i.e., normal ALT; (2) the immune-active or chronic hepatitis phase characterized by elevation in ALT level with declining serum viral DNA levels, presence of HBsAg and HBeAg in serum, active liver inflammation, and for most children, absence of overt clinical symptoms of infection; (3) the inactive HBsAg-carrier phase, characterized by undetectable HBeAg and presence of anti-HBe in serum, normal liver aminotransferase levels, low or absent levels of HBV DNA, and decreasing inflammation and fibrosis observed via liver histology; and (4) reactivation or e-antigen-negative chronic hepatitis B characterized by increased viral DNA levels, undetectable HBeAg, presence of anti-HBe, and normal or elevated ALT levels [14, 15]. Because a prolonged immune-active phase is correlated with development of chronic liver damage, cirrhosis, and/or HCC, medical practitioners must be vigilant in their monitoring of their HBV-infected patients and make prompt referral to a liver specialist when ALT and HBV DNA levels are elevated. Current therapies are effective only during the immune active phase. The goal of treatment is to prevent progressive liver scarring and to reduce the risk of HCC. This, in general, is achieved by reducing viral replication and decreasing inflammation. The treatment of pediatric patients with chronic HBV infection is best handled in partnership with a hepatologist or experienced pediatric infectious disease specialist.

All patients with chronic HBV infection should receive life-long management, regardless of ALT laboratory results, in order to monitor progression of liver disease and to assess the need for treatment and response to treatment. The frequency of and specific tests used for monitoring HBV infection are based on a constellation of factors including family history, phase of chronic HBV infection, and age of the patient. At a minimum, all patients need yearly testing. As stated previously, laboratory testing for monitoring purposes includes comprehensive HBV serologies, CBC, hepatic function panel, and periodic AFP (see Fig. 2). Ultrasound imaging is warranted at baseline for all children, regardless of age, to assess liver echotexture, nodules and masses, and spleen size. Among preteens and teenagers, ultrasound imaging should occur every 1–2 years. Liver biopsy may be used by the specialist to better assess the stage of the disease as an aid in decisions to treat.

Additional monitoring involves ongoing counseling and education for HBV-infected patients. Both the CDC and USA Public Health Service recommend prevention counseling for HBV-infected persons and the vaccination of household contacts and sexual partners. The primary care setting provides an opportunity for counseling HBsAg-positive persons and their family members on the ways to reduce the risk of transmitting the virus to others. Additionally, primary care providers are

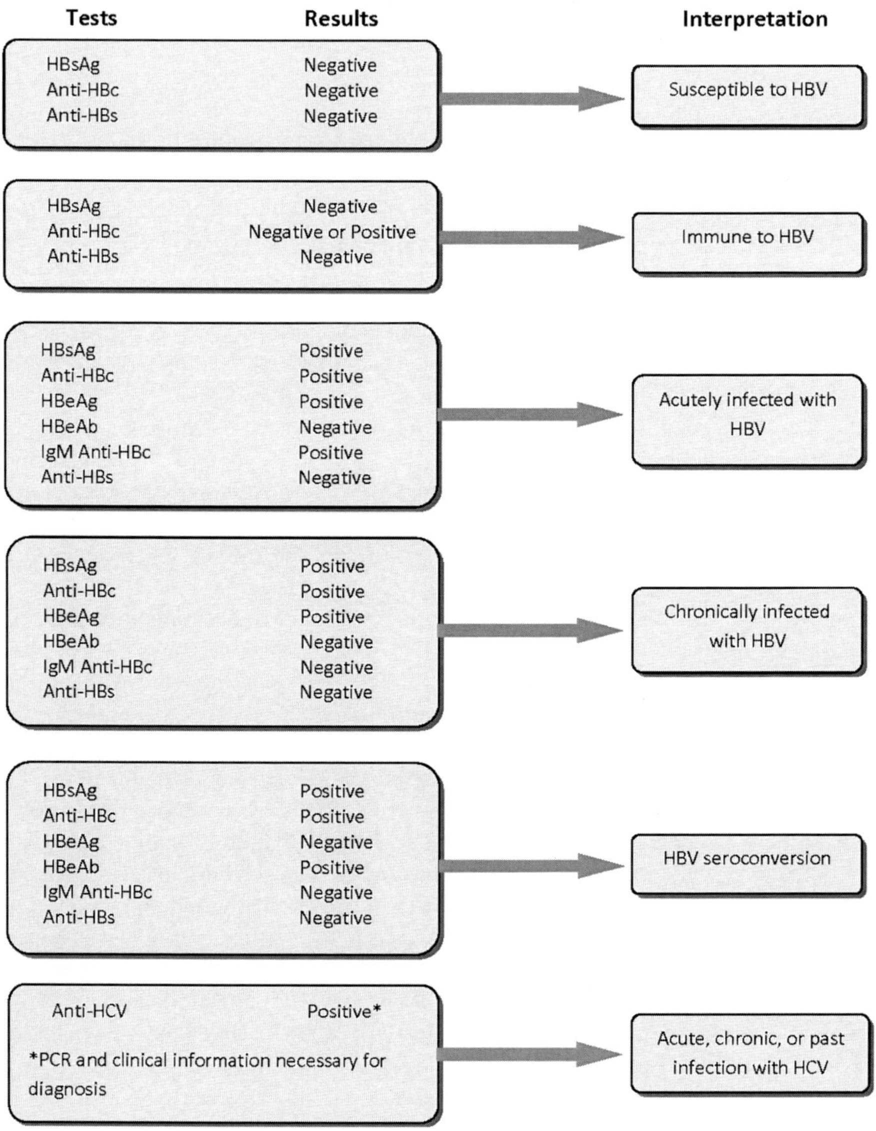

Fig. 2 Hepatitis B and C laboratory tests: interpretation of results

in a position to provide guidance to their patients to assuage some of the social concerns associated with chronic infection such as whom to tell, when to tell, and what legal protections are in place for preventing discrimination. Virus transmission prevention recommendations include [4] notification of household contacts; preventing the spread of infectious secretions or blood by covering open lesions and cuts; cleaning blood spills with appropriate disinfectants; refraining from sharing household items such as razors and toothbrushes; vaccination of previously unvaccinated adolescents and household contacts; and proper disposal of blood, bodily fluids, and medical waste. Among the teenage population with HBV infection, counseling should be provided regarding sexual and other risk behaviors, such as drinking alcohol and intravenous drug use. The CDC provides counseling recommendations for these populations on their website http://www.cdc.gov/hepatitis/B/PatientEduB.htm.

Hepatitis C

Natural History

Similar to hepatitis B, children with HCV often have no overt signs of infection. It is rare to develop jaundice even with an acute infection, and chronic infections are commonly asymptomatic until advanced liver disease has developed [16, 17]. The approach to hepatitis C has changed in the past decade due to our growing concern of the public health risk and because of the availability of new effective therapies for children. Among adults, hepatitis C is the leading cause for liver transplantation [18]. Accordingly, identification of HCV requires a pro-active approach including a heightened awareness on the part of the primary care practitioner and referral to a pediatric liver specialist, early in the course of the disease, for possible treatment.

HCV is the most common blood-borne infection and a significant infectious cause of chronic liver disease. In the USA, prevalence of chronic HCV infection is 1.8% [19]. Less is known about pediatric HCV infection compared with that in adults, due to the fact that only a small proportion of those infected with the virus are children. Among children in the USA, seroprevalence is 0.2% for those less than 12 years of age and 0.4% for those 12–19 years of age; however, the incidence of HCV may be greater due to the fact that many cases go undetected [20]. Diminishing the burden of pediatric HCV infection and HCV-related disease in the USA requires an increased understanding of appropriate methods of screening, monitoring, and management.

Transmission of HCV occurs through contaminated blood. Although the virus was discovered in 1989, blood products in the USA remained contaminated with hepatitis C until 1992 when effective anti-HCV screening tools were developed and implemented [16]. Prior to 1992, transfusion-acquired HCV was the most common mode of acquisition for the pediatric population. Presently, the risk of receiving HCV through blood products is less than one in a million [21]. In the USA, the most common pediatric groups to be infected include: children who have acquired the disease vertically from their mothers at the time of birth, children born outside of the contiguous USA who have had parenteral exposures, and children who have acquired the infection horizontally from close contacts or high-risk behaviors [19]. HCV infection, either acute or chronic, often goes undetected due to the lack of significant or distinct associated features of disease.

Hepatitis C is endemic in most regions of the world; however, there is considerable geographic diversity in the incidence and prevalence of infection. Countries with the highest reported prevalence rates are located in Africa and Asia, whereas areas with lower prevalence rates include industrialized nations in North America, northern and Western Europe, and Australia [8, 22]. Risk factors that commonly account for the majority of HCV transmission worldwide include blood transfusions from unscreened donors, intravenous drug use, and unsafe therapeutic injections [8]. Contaminated injection equipment is a major risk factor in many countries. In developing countries, an inadequate or non-existent supply of sterile syringes compounded by the administration of injections by non-professionals outside of medical settings contributes to the substantial risk and prevalence of HCV infection.

Six distinct HCV genotypes have been identified and vary in distribution throughout the world. In the USA genotypes 1, 2, and 3 are most common, with genotype 1 accounting for the majority of infections [23]. There is significant variation of HCV-related disease from patient to patient infected with similar HCV genotypes. Thus, HCV genotype is not utilized as a prognostic marker for HCV infection and predictor of disease outcome [24]. Rather, the determination of genotype has been identified as one parameter that could provide direction in the clinical management of chronic HCV infection.

In the USA, HCV infection in children is primarily caused by vertical transmission from mother to child during childbirth [25]. Perinatal or vertical transmission of HCV occurs with a transmission rate of approximately 5%, which increases to 22% in women with concomitant HIV infection [26, 27]. Because screening is not part of the maternal prenatal regimen, mothers who are unaware that they are infected may inadvertently transmit their infection to their children. Horizontal transmission of HCV infection among children can occur following exposure to infectious blood, accidental exposure to contaminated blood such as a needle stick, and from high-risk behaviors such as intravenous drug use and tattoos [20].

Prevention of HCV is problematic. There is no effective vaccination and post-exposure immunoglobulin is of no benefit [18, 28]. Furthermore, the asymptomatic presentation of HCV infection has contributed to gaps in the approach to screening for the infection. Therefore, it is necessary to be aware of specific groups of individuals who should receive particular attention for screening for HCV infection due to increased risk of acquisition (Table 3). As previously discussed, individuals with risk factors for HCV infection include intravenous drug users, children born to HCV-infected women (past or present infection), individuals with conditions associated with a high prevalence of HCV infection, such as HIV, and children born in regions with high HCV endemicity [18, 29]. Routine screening of these individuals will help control the burden of HCV infection.

Screening and Diagnosis

Screening and diagnostic methods have evolved from surrogate marker screening (e.g., elevated ALT) to antibody testing and, finally, to polymerase chain reaction (PCR) testing for viral RNA and genotype identification. Currently, two types of

Table 3 Persons who should be tested for HCV infection

Recommended populations for HCV testing
Intravenous drug: past, present, or one-time users
Individuals with medical conditions associated with a high prevalence of HCV infection
HIV infection
Hemodialysis (long-term use)
Elevated aminotransferase levels (ALT) otherwise unexplainable
Infants born to previously HCV-infected women
Recipients of transfusions and/or organ transplants prior to July 1992
Healthcare, emergency medical, and public safety workers after needle-stick, sharps, or mucosal exposures to HCV-positive blood
Sexual partners of HCV-positive individuals

tests are utilized to diagnose HCV infection – Enzyme Immunoassays (EIAs) to detect HCV antibodies and PCR tests to detect and quantify HCV RNA. EIAs, which determine the presence of HCV antibodies in the bloodstream, are most appropriate for initial testing for HCV because they are reproducible, inexpensive, and have high specificity and sensitivity [18, 30]. In the past, recombinant immunoblot assay (RIBA) was used, but the newer EIA is both more sensitive and more specific. Although EIAs have high specificity and sensitivity, positive HCV antibody results can indicate a resolved infection, an existing infection, or passively acquired antibodies. Therefore, qualitative and quantitative HCV RNA tests are useful in confirming viremia [24]. Qualitative HCV RNA tests are the more sensitive of the two tests and can detect as little as 100–1,000 copies per milliliter [31, 32]. Quantitative HCV PCR is utilized to provide information regarding viral load as it determines and quantifies the presence of active viremia. Although viral load does not directly correlate with disease progression or severity, it can aid in determining the probability of response to antiviral therapy [33, 34]. It is recommended that screening for HCV be performed with HCV antibody and if that returns positive, a qualitative PCR is obtained to determine if there is viremia. If there is a high suspicion for HCV, then PCR is often checked twice several weeks to months apart. The amount of virus detectable in the blood can fluctuate across the threshold of detection.

It is important to note that, at birth, children born to HCV-infected mothers will have antibodies in serum that have been passively acquired from the mothers [18]. Because this passive immunity may persist for up to 18 months, tests for HCV antibodies in children born to mothers with active infection should be administered after an infant has reached 12–15 months of age [18]. Tests prior to this time frame may result in "false-positive" results due to the presence of the mother's antibodies. Children who acquire the infection at birth from their mother are capable of spontaneous clearance, usually occurring within the first 2 years of life [35]. Therefore, it is advantageous to recheck HCV PCR around 24 months of age to confirm viremia. If the PCR is positive at 24 months of age, then referral to a specialist for consultation is recommended. Often treatment is not started at that time, but education from a provider skilled in the latest advances is advantageous. An important nonspecific laboratory test utilized to identify hepatic disease is the measurement of ALT and AST; however, these levels can be normal even when liver damage occurs as a result of HCV. Therefore, these laboratory chemistries should not be used as a screening tool, but rather are best used to assess risk of progression of HCV infection [36].

Medical Management of Chronic Infection

Once HCV infection is identified, management should be shared by a pediatric liver specialist and primary care practitioner. Treatment of chronic HCV infection in children can be effective, yet decisions regarding when to treat and whom to treat are often debated. Current therapies are lengthy and expensive, and have significant side effects. Furthermore, the risk of disease progression is low in the pediatric time frame. These negatives are weighed against our newer knowledge that children tolerate current therapies well and that treatment earlier in the course of the disease is more effective. Most recent pediatric studies demonstrate overall efficacy of therapy to be approximately 50% for those treated [37, 38] and significantly higher for genotypes 2 and 3 [32].

Although pediatric-specific management guidelines for chronic HCV infection have not been developed, universal medical management recommendations suggest that all patients with chronic HCV infection receive regular monitoring of liver disease before, during, and after treatment [20]. At initial assessment, laboratory testing includes a hepatic panel, CBC, and AFP. Ultrasound imaging is recommended as part of an initial evaluation in order to assess liver echotexture, nodules and masses, and spleen size [39]. Lastly, initial laboratory testings should also include assessment of viral genotype and viral load. This information is useful when discussing treatment options. Because it is now known that patients with less significant liver damage and a shorter duration of disease have an increased likelihood of responding to therapy, treatment should be considered for all patients at least 3 years of age with HCV. Referral to a specialist experienced in the management of HCV should occur early [18].

Genome sequencing has been instrumental in classifying HCV into unique genotypes. Viral genotyping is an essential early diagnostic step as it has been shown to aid in the understanding of the potential response to therapy and to determine length of treatment. There are six hepatitis C genotypes and more than 50 subtypes that vary in distribution throughout the world. Although whether specific genotypes influence the pathogenesis of liver disease or disease progression is uncertain, the impact on the response to anti-viral treatment is unquestionable – genotypes 2 and 3 have been associated with higher rates of response than genotype 1 or 4 [33, 34]. Thus, identifying the genotype is essential prior to discussions of therapy. Once identified, it is unnecessary to test for the genotype again as it does not change during the course of infection [30].

The goal of treatment is to prevent complications of HCV infection, which is primarily achieved by the eradication of the infection. Monitored by results of HCV

RNA testing, infection is considered to be eradicated when there is a sustained virologic response [16]. Nevertheless, therapies for HCV are still not completely effective, with "cure" rates in the range of 50% for genotypes 1 and 4, which accounts for the majority of patients [40]. To prevent other infections or a more serious form of hepatitis, children with chronic HCV infection should be vaccinated against hepatitis A and hepatitis B due to the increased risk for developing fulminant hepatitis if infected with either virus [18].

If the patient is not treated or has been treated and failed, on-going monitoring includes annual medical visits to monitor disease progression and determine appropriate course of action if treatment becomes warranted. Concomitant with medical monitoring, ongoing counseling and education for infected patients is central to the management of the HCV in order to prevent further transmission of the infection and should be provided in the primary care setting [19]. All patients with HCV should be considered infectious and informed of the possibility of transmission to others. Accordingly, physicians should communicate particular recommendations for reducing transmission, such as refraining from donating blood, organs, tissues, or semen as well as refraining from sharing household items such as razors and toothbrushes. Additionally, counseling should be provided to adolescents with HCV infection regarding sexual and other high-risk behaviors such as drinking alcohol and intravenous drug use.

Sexual transmission rates of HCV are minimal compared with that of HBV and HIV. It is recommended that individuals infected with HCV utilize barrier protection, such as condoms, when engaging in short-term sexual relationships due to the fact that the risk of transmission is approximately 1% per year [41]. The official recommendation from the CDC for monogamous relationships is that barrier methods of protection are not necessary because the risk is reduced to 0–0.6% per year [41]. However, the decision to use or not to use a barrier method is a personal decision a monogamous couple can make together.

Alcohol intake is a necessary topic to discuss with adolescents infected with HCV. Studies have demonstrated that alcohol consumption promotes the development and progression of fibrosis of the liver [42] and markedly expedites liver injury in individuals infected with HCV [43, 44]. Alcohol consumption, even moderately, exacerbates liver damage in HCV-infected individuals and, therefore, it is recommended that individuals with HCV abstain from alcohol use in order to deter further progression of the disease.

If a child embarks on treatment, the liver specialist closely monitors the child while he or she is on medication for side effects such as flu-like symptoms, fatigue, malaise, apathy, and cognitive changes. Although neutropenia may be marked, serious infections are very rare. Thyroid dysfunction is common, but most often transient. The benchmarks of successful treatment include loss of viremia at the end of treatment and sustained remission (negative PCR) 6 months later. For those who are no longer viremic 6 months after completing therapy, follow-up is moved to an annual basis. Studies for both adults and children have shown that the viral remission is durable for almost all who are virus negative 6 months after completion of treatment [45–47].

Several additional management areas are of concern when treating a child or adolescent with HCV. Obesity contributes to the progression of fibrosis in HCV-infected individuals and acts as an impediment to treatment [48]. Studies have demonstrated the impact of obesity on the rapid progression of fibrosis in patients with HCV [49, 50], and how, in one study, extreme obesity (BMI>30) contributed to a fourfold risk of HCC [51]. Therefore, it is recommended to counsel those who are overweight to lose weight in order to improve therapeutic response and overall health.

Other talking points typically covered by the physician focuses on the use of complementary medications and standard medications. Although the benefit of herbal remedies, such as silymarin (milk thistle), on chronic HCV infection has not been extensively studied, individuals with HCV frequently use this form of complementary medicine during the course of treatment [52]. Therefore, patients should seek advice from their physician prior to beginning a herbal regimen. The use of acetaminophen by children and adolescents with chronic HCV is warranted for short-term treatment (1–2 days) at age-appropriate doses. However, if the use is warranted for an extended period, consultation with a specialist is necessary in order to determine appropriate course.

No laws exist that protect individuals from discrimination based on the stigma associated with HCV infection status; however, several HCV discrimination cases that have been presented in court have been found to be covered under HIV discrimination litigation. Due to the possibility of the exposure of one's status, it is necessary for physicians to focus on providing appropriate education to individuals infected with HCV to equip them with the necessary information to convey to others in order to reduce the stigma surrounding the infection.

Active sports, such as soccer, field hockey, wrestling, basketball, and football, increase the potential for blood spills, which increases risk for exposure to HCV through infected blood. However, if standard precautions, as delineated by the AAP, are used by coaches, assistants, and student athletes, everyone has the opportunity to participate in organized sports. Therefore, education of the individual as it relates to appropriate precautions is necessary in order to reduce transmission [53].

Conclusion

In the USA, chronic HBV and HCV infections are still found in childhood as a result of gaps in screening and identification of infected individuals. Notwithstanding these gaps, our proficiency for managing and monitoring children with chronic viral infection has improved due largely to our increased understanding of the natural history and treatment of these infections. A more aggressive approach to identifying these children remains essential. Attention to those infected not only serves to limit the progression of HBV and HCV, but also addresses the general concern to prevent the spread of these infections. The primary care physician is in the unique position to identify and manage children with chronic viral hepatitis, thus improving long-term outcomes for these individuals while helping to reduce the global public health burden of these chronic infections.

References

1. Heron M. Deaths: leading causes for 2004. Natl Vital Stat Rep 2007;56:1–95.
2. Mathers CD, Bernard C, Iburg KM, Inoue M, Fate DM, Shibuya K. Global burden of disease in 2002: data sources, methods and results. World Health Organization 2003; 54.
3. Mast EE, Weinbaum CM, Fiore AE, et al. A comprehensive immunization strategy to eliminate transmission of hepatitis B virus infection in the United States: recommendations of the Advisory Committee on Immunization Practices (ACIP) Part II: immunization of adults. MMWR Recomm Rep 2006;55:1–33; quiz CE1–4.
4. Weinbaum CM, Williams I, Mast EE, et al. Recommendations for identification and public health management of persons with chronic hepatitis B virus infection. MMWR Recomm Rep 2008;57:1–20.
5. McMahon BJ, Alward WL, Hall DB, et al. Acute hepatitis B virus infection: relation of age to the clinical expression of disease and subsequent development of the carrier state. J Infect Dis 1985;151:599–603.
6. Hyams KC. Risks of chronicity following acute hepatitis B virus infection: a review. Clin Infect Dis 1995;20:992–1000.
7. Mast EE, Margolis HS, Fiore AE, et al. A comprehensive immunization strategy to eliminate transmission of hepatitis B virus infection in the United States: recommendations of the Advisory Committee on Immunization Practices (ACIP) part 1: immunization of infants, children, and adolescents. MMWR Recomm Rep 2005;54:1–31.
8. Shepard CW, Finelli L, Fiore AE, Bell BP. Epidemiology of hepatitis B and hepatitis B virus infection in United States children. Pediatr Infect Dis J 2005;24:755–60.
9. Zuckerman JN. Review: hepatitis B immune globulin for prevention of hepatitis B infection. J Med Virol 2007;79:919–21.
10. Hurie MB, Mast EE, Davis JP. Horizontal transmission of hepatitis B virus infection to United States-born children of Hmong refugees. Pediatrics 1992;89:269–73.
11. Mahoney FJ, Lawrence M, Scott C, Le Q, Lambert S, Farley TA. Continuing risk for hepatitis B virus transmission among Southeast Asian infants in Louisiana. Pediatrics 1995;96:1113–6.
12. Irwin GR, Allen AM, Bancroft WH, Karwacki JJ, Pinkerton RH, Russell PK. Hepatitis B antigen and antibody. Occurrence in families of asymptomatic HB AG carriers. JAMA 1974; 227:1042–3.
13. Chakravarty R, Chowdhury A, Chaudhuri S, et al. Hepatitis B infection in Eastern Indian families: need for screening of adult siblings and mothers of adult index cases. Public Health 2005;119:647–54.
14. Haber BA, Block JM, Jonas MM, et al. Recommendations for screening, monitoring, and referral of pediatric chronic hepatitis B. Pediatrics 2009;124:e1007–13.
15. Hoofnagle JH, Doo E, Liang TJ, Fleischer R, Lok AS. Management of hepatitis B: summary of a clinical research workshop. Hepatology 2007;45:1056–75.
16. Jonas MM. Children with hepatitis C. Hepatology 2002;36:S173–8.
17. Mast EE, Alter MJ, Margolis HS. Strategies to prevent and control hepatitis B and C virus infections: a global perspective. Vaccine 1999;17:1730–3.
18. Hepatitis C. In: Red Book; 2009. p. 357–60.
19. Alter MJ. Prevention of spread of hepatitis C. Hepatology 2002;36:S93–8.
20. American Academy of Pediatrics. Hepatitis C virus infection. Committee on infectious diseases. In: Pediatrics; 1998. p. 481–5.
21. Hillyer CD, Josephson CD, Blajchman MA, Vostal JG, Epstein JS, Goodman JL. Bacterial contamination of blood components: risks, strategies, and regulation: joint ASH and AABB educational session in transfusion medicine. Hematology Am Soc Hematol Educ Program 2003:575–89.
22. Wasley A, Alter MJ. Epidemiology of hepatitis C: geographic differences and temporal trends. Semin Liver Dis 2000;20:1–16.
23. Hnatyszyn HJ. Chronic hepatitis C and genotyping: the clinical significance of determining HCV genotypes. Antivir Ther 2005;10:1–11.

24. Pawlotsky JM. Use and interpretation of virological tests for hepatitis C. Hepatology 2002;36:S65–73.
25. Roberts EA, Yeung L. Maternal-infant transmission of hepatitis C virus infection. Hepatology 2002;36:S106–13.
26. Yeung LT, King SM, Roberts EA. Mother-to-infant transmission of hepatitis C virus. Hepatology 2001;34:223–9.
27. Zanetti AR, Tanzi E, Newell ML. Mother-to-infant transmission of hepatitis C virus. J Hepatol 1999;31 (Suppl 1):96–100.
28. Krawczynski K, Alter MJ, Tankersley DL, et al. Effect of immune globulin on the prevention of experimental hepatitis C virus infection. J Infect Dis 1996;173:822–8.
29. Strader DB, Wright T, Thomas DL, Seeff LB. Diagnosis, management, and treatment of hepatitis C. Hepatology 2004;39:1147–71.
30. Lauer GM, Walker BD. Hepatitis C virus infection. N Engl J Med 2001;345:41–52.
31. Fried MW. Diagnostic testing for hepatitis C: practical considerations. Am J Med 1999;107: 31S–5S.
32. National Institutes of Health Consensus Development Conference Statement: Management of hepatitis C 2002 (June 10–12, 2002). Gastroenterology 2002;123(6):2082–99.
33. Poynard T, Marcellin P, Lee SS, et al. Randomised trial of interferon alpha2b plus ribavirin for 48 weeks or for 24 weeks versus interferon alpha2b plus placebo for 48 weeks for treatment of chronic infection with hepatitis C virus. International Hepatitis Interventional Therapy Group (IHIT). Lancet 1998;352:1426–32.
34. McHutchison JG, Gordon SC, Schiff ER, et al. Interferon alfa-2b alone or in combination with ribavirin as initial treatment for chronic hepatitis C. Hepatitis Interventional Therapy Group. N Engl J Med 1998;339:1485–92.
35. Ceci O, Margiotta M, Marello F, et al. High rate of spontaneous viral clearance in a cohort of vertically infected hepatitis C virus infants: what lies behind? J Hepatol 2001;35:687–8.
36. National Institutes of Health Consensus Development Conference Panel statement: management of hepatitis C. Hepatology 1997;26:2S–10S.
37. Jara P, Hierro L, de la Vega A, et al. Efficacy and safety of peginterferon-alpha2b and ribavirin combination therapy in children with chronic hepatitis C infection. Pediatr Infect Dis J 2008; 27:142–8.
38. Schwarz KB, Gonzalez-Peralta RP, Murray KF, et al. Peginterferon with or without ribavirin for chronic Hepatitis C in children and adolescents: final results of the PEDS-C trial. Hepatology 2008;48:418A.
39. Fontana RJ, Lok AS. Noninvasive monitoring of patients with chronic hepatitis C. Hepatology 2002;36:S57–64.
40. Roache K, Haber B. Hepatitis C Virus infection. Pediatric Eastroenterology Board Review Manual 2007; Volume 1, Part 3:2–9.
41. CDC. Recommendations for prevention and control of Hepatitis C Virus (HCV) infection and HCV-related chronic disease. MMWR Recomm Rep. 1998;47:1–39.
42. Poynard T, Bedossa P, Opolon P. Natural history of liver fibrosis progression in patients with chronic hepatitis C. The OBSVIRC, METAVIR, CLINIVIR, and DOSVIRC groups. Lancet 1997;349:825–32.
43. Harris DR, Gonin R, Alter HJ, et al. The relationship of acute transfusion-associated hepatitis to the development of cirrhosis in the presence of alcohol abuse. Ann Intern Med 2001;134: 120–4.
44. Wiley TE, McCarthy M, Breidi L, Layden TJ. Impact of alcohol on the histological and clinical progression of hepatitis C infection. Hepatology 1998;28:805–9.
45. Kelly D, Haber B, Gonzalez-Peralta RP, et al. Sustained virologic response to interferon alfa-2b plus ribavirin predicts long-term clearance of HCV in pediatric patients at 5 year follow-up. J Hepatol 2008;48:S298–9.
46. Lindsay K, Manns MP, Gordon SC, et al. S1001 Clearance of HCV at 5 year follow-up for peginterferon alfa-2b ± ribavirin is predicted by sustained virologic response at 24 weeks post treatment. Gastroenterology 2008;134:A-772.

47. Maylin S, Martinot-Peignoux M, Moucari R, et al. Eradication of hepatitis C virus in patients successfully treate for chronic hepatitis C. Gastroenterology 2008;135:821–9.
48. Ghany MG, Strader DB, Thomas DL, Seeff LB. Diagnosis, management, and treatment of hepatitis C: an update. Hepatology 2009;49:1335–74.
49. Hourigan LF, Macdonald GA, Purdie D, et al. Fibrosis in chronic hepatitis C correlates significantly with body mass index and steatosis. Hepatology 1999;29:1215–9.
50. Ortiz V, Berenguer M, Rayon JM, Carrasco D, Berenguer J. Contribution of obesity to hepatitis C-related fibrosis progression. Am J Gastroenterol 2002;97:2408–14.
51. Chen CL, Yang HI, Yang WS, et al. Metabolic factors and risk of hepatocellular carcinoma by chronic hepatitis B/C infection: a follow-up study in Taiwan. Gastroenterology 2008; 135:111–21.
52. Seeff LB, Lindsay KL, Bacon BR, Kresina TF, Hoofnagle JH. Complementary and alternative medicine in chronic liver disease. Hepatology 2001;34:595–603.
53. Kukka C. Bloodborne infections: should they be disclosed? Is differential treatment necessary? J Sch Nurs 2004;20:324–30.

Index

MIX
Papier aus verantwortungsvollen Quellen
Paper from responsible sources
FSC® C105338

Printed by Books on Demand, Germany